Quit Stalling on Malaria Vaccines, and Other Ideas for Combating Malaria

by
Michael Fullerton

Dedicated to my wife, Mary, who has done a tremendous number of great things for me, which recently includes the cooking of many pans of excellent cornbread. God bless her.

Table of Contents

Introduction

After reading lots of scholarly articles about malaria, one of the world's major killers, the main impression I get is that by now there should be at least one malaria vaccine available for anyone who wants it. Another impression I get is that if people were better educated in general and especially about malaria, many fewer people would die of the disease. Another idea that comes to me is that the medicines to treat malaria should be free so that people wouldn't try to save money by hoping that the disease that their child has isn't severe and that the kid will be fine in a couple days and the family will have saved some cash. We're spending money on stupid things and not spending money to save people's lives. A few days ago the United States government grounded a fighter jet, the F-35, because it's too dangerous for pilots. They don't know what's wrong with it. The price for this piece of junk has been over $400 billion. You could pay for a lot of free medicine with that.

Here's a quote from the New York Times from August of 1984: "Federal officials announced today that scientists have cleared the last major hurdle to development of a vaccine against malaria..." M. Peter McPherson, administrator of the Agency for International Development, expected that a vaccine would be ready for trial in humans within 12 to 18 months and widely available throughout the world within five years. So at least somebody thought a vaccine should have been ready by 1989, 25 years ago as I write this.

McPherson was right. There should have been. I think one of the problems is that scientists and officials aimed too high. They wanted a vaccine that would be super-effective, like preventing 95% of cases of the disease, and they refused to settle for anything less. Back in the 1970s researchers used live attenuated Plasmodium falciparum parasites to vaccinate some volunteers. A short time later they were exposed to potentially pathogenic Plasmodium falciparum and did not get the disease. It

1

seemed that they'd discovered a super-effective malaria vaccine, and they had, in the short run anyway. But those live attenuated bugs were difficult to produce and use as a vaccine. So most researchers decided to try making an easier vaccine to produce. Not a bad idea, but the live vaccine spoiled them for anything that wasn't as effective. At some point early on someone in charge should have said, "OK, we still haven't got the totally ass-kickin' malaria vaccine yet, but we should get something out there, to the masses, that is at least somewhat effective." But nobody ever did, even though effective vaccines and good ideas for vaccines have been around for a long time.

No question malaria is a deadly disease, from half a million to 1.5 million die from it every year, depending on your source, mostly young children in tropical or almost tropical countries, especially sub-Saharan Africa, but also in India, Southeast Asia, the tropical parts of the Americas. Most people who get the most deadly kind of malaria, Plasmodium falciparum, don't die. It seems that some people in Africa don't consider malaria a big problem. I suspect these are people who have had it, maybe a number of times, and they survived, and they know lots of people who survived their bouts of malaria. For them it's like, "What's the big deal?" The deal is, there are many children who are healthy, enjoying life with a big possible happy future ahead of them who are suddenly killed by Plasmodium falciparum malaria. Not only that, there are many more who have long-term neurological problems because they had a bad case of cerebral malaria, also caused by Plasmodium falciparum. Either way, death or bran damage, it's a rotten thing to happen to a young child, especially when many cases of the disease could be prevented or made less severe. These goals are attainable right now, with the science we have presently available.

Of course it's not just children who die of malaria. A writer who's lived in Africa a long time as a photo-safari guide, Mark C. Ross, says, "If you live in Africa you see human death. I encounter a dead body somewhere here on an almost weekly basis. Some have died sad, slow, and painful deaths bathed in malarial sweat. Another death might have been the bloody and anachronistic killing of a poor street thief who stole a ten dollar necklace, was caught, and then beaten to death on the spot (1)." Ross stays in Africa because he loves the animals. He's originally from Indiana. The most dangerous animals that Ross encountered seem to have been humans. Some of his clients, who were also his friends, were killed by a group of rebels. Ross and his group were looking for gorillas. Ross says he still doesn't sleep well and it happened years ago. I would think walking by people dying or dead from malaria regularly might keep you up at night, wondering if there isn't a way to prevent it. I think there is, in many cases.

Malaria is transmitted by Anopheles mosquitoes to humans. The mosquitoes get P. Falciparum parasites from humans. So if you cut down on the cases of malaria that in itself might help to cut cases of the disease even further because fewer of the mosquitoes will get the P. Falciparum when they bite people.

A recent study from Burkina Faso, a small country in sub-Saharan Africa, finds lots of malaria among children 0-5 years old. The authors followed 555 children for a year and found that during that time 86.2% of them got at least one case of malaria (3). Some got it 6 times. So it seems that in that part of the world, if you're a young child, with current practices you're probably going to catch malaria at least once a year. The authors don't mention if any of their subjects died or suffered brain-damaging cerebral malaria. The authors do mention that among the youngest children in their study, kids from 0-2 years old, over 90% of them got malaria. They suggest that the youngest group would be the best targets for malaria vaccines. Seems like a good idea, but too young and antibodies in the child's blood from the mother might react with the vaccine to make it useless.

Maybe the official arbiters of science over the years have been waiting for the perfect malaria vaccine because they're afraid if they make a less than super-effective vaccine available it will make them look bad. I'll tell you what looks bad is governments and scientific bureaucracies not making some kind of malaria vaccine available right now. There are many different malaria vaccines that have been shown to have strong anti-malarial effects in animals and some in humans too. Even non-malarial vaccines such as one for tuberculosis, the BCG vaccine, and the yellow fever vaccine have shown anti-malarial effects in humans, apparently by stimulating the non-specific immune system. We'll get to more about this later. So take the BCG vaccine and throw some malarial proteins in with it, do a round or so of testing and get it out there.

There are definitely other good possibilities for vaccines, like GlaxoSmithKline's RTS,S vaccine, which has been dragged through many years of trials in the hopes they could get absolute prevention of the disease up toward some lofty above-50% level. But even if the vaccine doesn't prevent someone from getting the disease it might make the disease less severe by giving the immune system a head start on fighting the parasites. It's likely that this head start would save lives. It's a crime that at least some kind of vaccine is not yet available for malaria.

Most of the people who die from it are in poor countries and have dark-colored skin. Maybe racism is partly to blame for the ridiculously long time it's taken the top bosses of the governmental organizations that regulate science and drug companies to make a malaria vaccine available. This racism might be unintentional, carried out by people who don't consider themselves racist at all. Researchers have found unconscious racial bias in a number of studies. Maybe that's what's happening. On the other hand, there are still people in the world who are consciously racist.

Maybe there are people in powerful positions in developed countries, like the United States, who don't mind if the countries of sub-Saharan Africa are somewhat crippled by tropical diseases, making those places easier to exploit by the more "civilized" countries of the north. I hope that's not happening, but you never know. The U.S. has a cold-blooded federal government that starts wars regularly. Some call it "regime change", but it's war.

The BCG vaccine for tuberculosis has never been close to 100% effective at preventing tuberculosis, in fact sometimes it prevents very few cases, yet it's been available for over 70 years, and has saved millions of lives. It's time to get at least one malaria vaccine to the public. RTS,S will probably be the first. But don't stop there. There are many excellent ideas for malaria vaccines. It's time to streamline the approval process for malaria vaccines. A malaria vaccine candidate shouldn't be considered garbage just because it doesn't prevent the disease in over 30% of those who are vaccinated. Any degree of immunity elicited by the vaccine might be enough to save a person's life or keep them from suffering life-altering brain damage. Long-term follow-up might be the best way to assess which vaccine is best, and even then the results might be difficult to interpret. Get some vaccines out there at prices people can afford, or better yet, for free. Having a number of different malaria vaccines might be similar to the way that people become more or less immune to the disease over a number of years and a number of malaria infections.

A recent article from *Malaria Journal* says that the severity of malaria is determined by the species of Plasmodium, immune status of the patient, prior use of chemoprophylaxis, and the timeliness and type of treatment given (4). Immune status is a big one. If you've had a number of cases of malaria already there's a better chance that your immune system will recognize and destroy the parasites than if your immune system has never been exposed to it. This is probably why the younger children are at greater risk of suffering severe or deadly malaria than older people in the same area, because the older folks have developed some immunity.

The authors say that 1 million children die each year from malaria. They also mention that about 150 international travelers die each year after spending time in countries where malaria is common. Two fatalities among travelers that the authors examined were people who hadn't taken chemoprophylaxis. They also found that people taking chemoprophylaxis had fewer parasites when they did get malaria. Higher parasite burden has been linked to worse outcome. The authors stress that travelers, who often have no immunity to malaria at all, who are like the youngest children in that respect, have to be careful to take the anti-malarial drugs on schedule, or risk a bad case of malaria. They also noted that advanced age was associated with worse outcome for travelers who got malaria. So it seems that if you've never been exposed to malaria you're better off getting it as a child than as an old adult. Perhaps the child's innate immune system is better at fighting malaria than the older adult's. The authors mention that African travelers in Africa tend to have less severe cases of malaria, probably because they already have some immunity to it.

 The idea of a vaccine or vaccines for malaria is to give people's immune systems exposure to the disease without actually giving them the disease. There's a huge number of parasite proteins to choose from. Of course you want the best ones but you don't want to spend any more years splitting hairs or searching for perfection. Get something out there and worry about perfection later. You wonder why malaria has been such a difficult disease to get a super-effective vaccine for. It's probably at least partly because the parasite goes through a number of stages during its life where it changes dramatically, including its parasite proteins. The immune system just starts to zero in on the parasite at one stage of its life when it suddenly changes and the immune system no longer recognizes it. The parasites multiply fast. Very quickly you have huge numbers of unrecognizable parasites in your blood. Plasmodium falciparum itself has a lot of genetic diversity. Just because you're immune to one strain of the bug doesn't mean another strain of P. falciparum can't make you sick because its proteins are a little different.

Nevertheless, there are some parasitic proteins that are largely conserved, which are probably the best ones to use for vaccines. And the evidence is that after enough exposures to the disease, people tend to get immune to it. This happens with age, which is encouraging because it means that vaccines should do some good, even if they don't make the person completely immune, which is apparently what the big honchos in science have been holding out for.

Vaccines

The authors in an article from 2012, Moorthy et al., state that the RTS,S/AS01 vaccine should be ready for general use and approval by African countries in 2015 (5). They say that "on average the vaccine reduces the frequency of new infections by 50%." That sounds great! It's not perfect, but it's a big improvement over no vaccine at all. They want to vaccinate at somewhere between 6 and 14 weeks of age, in three doses about the same time as a bunch of other vaccines are given. One wonders how many people will go along with the three-dose plan. I can picture many giving their kids one dose, which might not keep as many children from getting malaria, but might still reduce the severity of the disease for most who get it, probably enough to save some lives.

What's more, in areas where malaria is endemic, children will probably receive some antibodies to malaria from their mothers at birth. These antibodies usually last from 6 to 9 months; children who get them are often protected from getting malaria for the first 3-6 months of life (6). This means the antibodies are fairly strong. I would guess that vaccinating kids for malaria whose mothers have had malaria should be done later than 9 months, otherwise you might be wasting vaccine, not to mention the time and effort of the people involved. If passively acquired antibodies from the mother latch onto malarial antigens in the vaccine it probably won't give the child's immune system time to process that antigen and remember it for later.

Some people here in the U.S. think that vaccinations can cause autism. Some researchers have rejected this notion, but scientists have been wrong before. There are people who insist that their children were doing great shortly before they received routine vaccinations, after which the children became withdrawn and ultimately were diagnosed with autism. Given the ever-increasing load of vaccines inflicted on children, some at very early ages, one can picture autoimmune mishaps where the immune system, suddenly faced with a load of foreign antigens and adjuvants, attacks the child's neurons. In order to avoid this, maybe it would be better to wait beyond 14 weeks for the malaria vaccine to be given, like maybe 9 months. Children who drink mother's milk are protected from malaria to some extent anyway, although this protection from is not specific to malaria. It's a general immune boost, which it would be best if all children had. This later date for the malaria vaccine might cut down on severe reactions to the vaccine, especially if the vaccine is no longer given at the same time as other vaccines. We'll get into more about severe reactions to RTS,S shortly. If there's a good chance maternally acquired antimalarial antibodies will disable the vaccine before 9 months anyway, why bother with it till then?

Moorthy et al. state that insecticide-treated bed nets greatly reduce malaria transmission. Unfortunately, many people in Africa don't use them. We'll get into this more later. In some cases, only a small fraction of people use them. Education seems to be one of the key ways to fight malaria. What I can picture is having the baby sleep under a net for quite a while, like 9 months, until the kid's immune system matures, and then give her the vaccine. If you insist on the three shots, spread them out over time, like more than several weeks apart. Several months might be safer.

The authors' main question in this article is cost-effectiveness, which they seem to equate with keeping the person from getting the disease for a certain amount of time. This is a good goal, but how about the goal of keeping children from dying from malaria or suffering long-term neurological damage from it? The authors seem to think that if the vaccine does not prevent the disease it has failed, when in reality, it might still be working well enough to save the child's life. The authors question the duration of protection while talking about cost-effectiveness. Their version of protection is protection from ever getting the disease. How about protection from death by the disease or long-term brain problems from it? The authors conclude that more research into "cost-effectiveness" is needed. I don't think the question of cost effectiveness in regard to malaria is cost effective. Get a good vaccine ready to go and ramp up production so that it's cheap enough for everyone to afford. Let individuals judge whether it's cost effective for them and their children.

Even if they do get around to approving the RTS,S vaccine, there will be proposals for different malaria vaccines because the RTS,S isn't close to perfect. Another recent article suggests using erythrocyte-binding antigen 175 (EBA-175) as part of a vaccine. The authors found that when they induced antibodies to this part of the P. falciparum parasite that the parasites were usually blocked from entering red blood cells through a common type of receptor (6). Entering red blood cells is necessary for one of the parasite's main stages of life. If they can't get into the red blood cells, they're screwed. Unfortunately in real life the parasite has multiple ways of entering the RBC. The authors of this study eliminated the other entryways to show that EBA-175 is definitely a way that the parasite can enter RBCs. They also note that antibodies to one EBA-175 worked well for a number of different types of P. falciparum parasites.

The authors are not claiming that they have a ready-to-go vaccine. They're just saying that the EBA-175 should be considered as part of a vaccine that would include other parasitic proteins that enable them to enter RBCs. If you could keep the bugs out of the blood cells, you've beaten them. The authors say right up front that, "P. falciparum has redundant ligands that mediate invasion of erythrocytes." They mention that Plasmodium vivax used to be the most common kind of malaria in Africa. P. vivax requires Duffy blood group receptors for invasion of RBCs. P. vivax doesn't have multiple entryways like P. falciparum does. People in Africa have lost Duffy blood group proteins through evolution, largely eliminating P. vivax in Africa. Maybe P. falciparum is an evolutionary descendant of P. vivax, a descendant that has still managed to stay alive in Africa, thrive actually.

The authors note that EBA-175 forms rosettes with RBCs more than other P. falciparum ligands. Rosettes are bad. That's when RBCs latch onto each other. Rosetting has been linked to more severe disease and cerebral malaria. The rosettes can clog small blood vessels, which can cause the death of cells that rely on those vessels, including brain cells. If you can keep RBCs from rosetting, that's great, but there is more than one way for rosetting to happen. Even so, this makes EBA-175 a more attractive candidate for inclusion in a vaccine. You could probably save some lives with just an EBA-175 vaccine, but it wouldn't be perfect. The authors also note that naturally acquired antibodies to EBA-175 are found in people who live in malaria endemic places. Having these antibodies is surely good for them. For the time being, put out an EBA-175 vaccine.

The next article tells about pre-erythrocyte vaccines and a lot about malaria in general. Pre-erythrocyte means that they want to kill the parasites before they invade red blood cells. The authors figure this gives them about a week and it's at a time when there aren't many parasites you need to kill (7). Here's how malaria usually progresses: The mosquito bites you and you receive some malaria parasites in your skin. The authors say from a few dozen to a few hundred, which are pretty small numbers, when you're talking about something that small. The parasites, called sporozoites at this stage, can migrate through cells, which they do, until they reach a blood vessel. They float around until they reach the liver. Then they migrate through liver cells until they find the kind they want.

Once inside a liver cell they like they expand and multiply, making tens of thousands of merozoites, according to the authors. The merozoites eventually break out of the liver cell and infect red blood cells. The infection of RBCs is when the symptoms of malaria begin and the pre-erythrocytic stage ends.

Even if the immune system with the help of a vaccine is able to kill 90% of the sporozoites you're still going to have tens of thousands of merozoites to infect your RBCs in a week, so you'll probably have symptoms of the disease, and the vaccine, by what seem to be the prevailing standards, will be deemed a failure. But the fact is, there could have been way more merozoites ravaging your blood cells, which probably would have made the disease much more severe, maybe even deadly. So maybe the vaccine wasn't a failure after all.

One of the reasons you can get malaria a bunch of times is because the sporozoites themselves don't cause disease symptoms. They seem to float around not doing much harm, so the immune system doesn't develop a strong resistance to them. It's after they turn into merozoites when the trouble starts. So the authors idea is to make the immune system resistant to the sporozoites so they can never give rise to their exceedingly nasty and numerous descendants, the merozoites. The problem is that it's difficult to get the immune system worked up about something when there's no disease symptoms. The immune system doesn't make the connection between sporozoites and merozoites, or at least not as strongly as one would hope.

The authors say "infections with sporozoites do not usually confer highly effective PE (pre-erythrocytic) immunity in naturally infected humans or in

11

experimentally infected rodents." Although people do seem to become immune to malaria to varying degrees, probably depending on exposure. The more exposure the more immune. Maybe it would take a number of vaccinations for a person to become immune to the disease with a pre-erythrocytic vaccine such as the RTS,S. The researchers who have developed the vaccine recommend three shots early in life and maybe more later.

Unfortunately the RTS,S vaccine was originally preserved in thimerosal, which contains mercury, according to the authors. For any vaccine, thimerosal is bad, but it's especially bad for vaccines that require a number of shots. It's unacceptable. Mercury is a neurotoxic poison and may have caused some vaccinated children to become autistic. Hopefully, the RTS,S vaccine that is eventually put on the market will not use thimerosal as a preservative.

One of the reasons the authors and many others are still optimistic about a pre-erythrocytic vaccine is that, "sterile protection develops in mice, non-human primates and humans following immunization with radiation attenuated sporozoites." Sterile protection means you don't get the disease symptoms at all, your immune system wipes it out that early. The authors say that both antibodies and T-cells are involved in this protection. The antibodies latch onto sporozoites before they reach liver cells and T-cells destroy infected liver cells. No massive load of merozoites in your bloodstream.

The authors note that the circumsporozoite protein (CSP), which is what the RTS,S vaccine targets, does not have to be present on the radiation attenuated sporozoites in order for those sporozoites to be effective at inducing sterile protection. This has been tested using genetically altered sporozoites that didn't have CSP. This is evidence in favor of the authors' idea of checking more of the thousands of other proteins P. falciparum has for vaccine making. The authors say that P. faliparum has over 5300 expressed genes but only four genes are currently in use for vaccine development. That's hardly any. The authors suggest that we come up with some kind of process for evaluating genes for vaccines, to get the best genes for the immune system to zero in on. The best might be genes that are highly conserved among all types of P. falciparum and the other less deadly types of malaria also. But it might also help to put a lot of them in one vaccine so the immune system might have many targets instead of just one or a few. After all, if you get the whole sporozoite your immune system can learn to recognize a lot of antigens, not just one.

The odd thing about radiation attenuated sporozoites' ability to induce such a strong immunity is that the actual disease doesn't give you much immunity to sporozoites even though your immune system has had access to them. Maybe the immune system forgets the non-attenuated sporozoites to a large extent because of the symptomatic disease caused by merozoites that comes a short time afterward. Maybe the immune system judges the merozoite invasion to be much more dangerous and so dedicates a lot more of its resources to that and away from the recent sporozoites. Who knows? Maybe there's a chemical that merozoites produce that represses the immune system, including its responses to sporozoites.

The authors say that circumsporozoite protein vaccines didn't work well at preventing malaria until RTS,S. But at first RTS,S didn't work well either until they tried some different adjuvants, which are concoctions that are designed to boost the immune response that are included with the vaccine. The authors tell us the RTS,S researchers got lucky once and 6 out of 7 volunteers who were given the malaria parasites were protected from getting the disease (85%). They couldn't get that percentage later. Researchers got 32-50% protection depending on the adjuvant and the authors don't say how long it lasted. But I would guess that the people who got the vaccine but still contracted malaria got a less severe disease. Who knows? Maybe the 6 out of 7 volunteers were all well past 9 months of age and didn't have to worry about maternal antibodies ruining the effect of their malaria vaccine.

In the vaccine trial as soon as those vaccinated got the disease they were given drugs to get rid of it, so it's hard to say how severe it would have been. But it's likely that fewer sporozoites were able to give rise to merozoites because a number of sporozoites had been targeted by the immune system. The latest figures for RTS,S that the authors quote are around 50% sterile protection for 13 months for the first vaccination, which sounds great. Once again, most of those that didn't get sterile protection probably got some protection.

Earlier I guessed that if a vaccine added more malarial antigens it might be better. The authors mention one, the ME-TRAP vaccine, which had 5 antigens in addition to the CSP. It was a failure in terms of sterile protection. Still, I'm guessing that if it were given to a lot of people, it would save lives and reduce malaria-caused brain problems. Maybe the designers of ME-TRAP have a good idea that actually works to keep people alive and healthy, but doesn't prevent the disease entirely in a high percentage of cases. I wouldn't give up on the idea of using multiple antigens on a vaccine. After all, that's what you get with the radiation attenuated sporozoites (RAS), lots of antigens, which have given high levels of sterile protection in the past. Apparently one of the drawbacks of RAS is that you need many of them for the vaccine to work. Maybe the ME-TRAP researchers need to boost the dose.

You might be thinking, "Hey! If the RAS vaccine works so well, why not just go with that?" The authors say whole sporozoite vaccines are being worked on. They mention an RAS vaccine that was given subcutaneously or intradermally that had "poor efficacy". It seems that earlier RAS vaccines were given by way of mosquito bites, lots of them, maybe 1000, according to the authors.

They also mention genetically altered parasites for vaccines, sporozoites that would stop developing before the merozoite stage, but add that there are problems making the genetically altered parasites so far. The authors are optimistic about a plan to inoculate people with regular disease-causing sporozoites and then kill them off with chloroquine before patients get disease symptoms. It seems to give high levels of sterile protection that lasts for 28 months. The authors say it would require fewer sporozoites which would make it easier to produce. Even so, you have to keep the parasites alive and make sure they don't become immune to the chloroquine. Genetic mutations happen fast in these small creatures.

If you could just get a good dead vaccine, it would be easier. The authors seem to agree. They note that the sporozoite uses about 2000 genes, 41 of which are exclusive to them. Let's add some antigens onto the RTS,S. It seems like a good idea to me. If RTS,S uses only the CSP and its approved for general use, it may give rise to sporozoites that don't have the CSP. A vaccine that targets that protein would definitely push the P. falciparum population in that direction. So add some antigens to the RTS,S.

The authors have a section titled "Downselecting PE (pre-erythrocytic) antigens as vaccine candidates." So out of 2000 or so genes they're trying to figure out the best ones for a vaccine. They say that 19 antigens were found to be strongly associated with RAS-induced immunity. So how about a vaccine with all 19 antigens? The authors don't say anything about that, but they do mention a process where some researchers evaluated 34 antigens with high levels of transcription, in other words, the parasite uses those genes a lot. They whittled that list down to 3 antigens which were found to not be protective at all for mice. Why not try a vaccine with all 34 of the original high transcription antigens? I suppose it's more difficult to make copies of all those antigens rather than just 3, but if the 34 antigen vaccine works then you've got something. On the other hand, my hunch is that even if the mice who got the 3-antigen vaccine weren't protected from getting the disease, they probably got some protection from death or brain damage due to severe disease.

The authors say that in a different study a large fraction of rodents received sterile immunity from a 3-

antigen vaccine. It sounds like a good vaccine as is, but maybe a few more antigens would make it better.

The authors talk about various adjuvants and vectors. Adjuvants, as you recall, are things added to the vaccine that enhance immune response. Vectors are ways of delivering the vaccine that can have immune stimulating effects, such as putting the vaccine on a virus. Immune systems tend to take viruses very seriously and mount a stronger defense to them than just some inert liquids. The authors mention a vaccine that used a pox virus vector that contained 7 proteins, 2 from the sporozoite stage, 1 from the liver stage, 3 from the blood stage, and 1 from the sexual stage of P falciparum's life cycle. This sounds like a great vaccine. The immune system has a head start on every one of those tricky stages, the stages that make the little beast such a killer. If you're one of those that gets the vaccine but still winds up getting the disease the vaccine will likely help you have an easier time of it. Because let's face it, the blood stage is where the disease can kill you. To have a vaccine targeting 3 antigens at this stage is a great idea. If the disease has to progress to this stage for people, you want some protection here too. So far the RTS,S only prevents about 50% of cases of the disease. That's a lot of people who will still get sick. An antigen for the sexual stage seems good too if it works to keep the parasites from multiplying. This 7 antigens from all stages of parasite development vaccine seems like a refreshing realization that you might not ever get a perfect malaria vaccine, one that prevents the disease in all people, or even close to it. Instead, let's prevent as many cases as we can and for the rest, make the disease as mild and survivable as possible.

The authors in the next study tried out RTS,S on a group of 170 children in Tanzania. They had a similar sized control group. The RTS,S/AS02D formulation was used which contains a hepatitis B antigen and is specially made for children, which the authors figure might give the kids some resistance to hepatitis B (8). The authors mention that a group of kids 1-4 years old in Gambia were protected for 18 months against "clinical malaria and severe disease." One wonders if we're talking about severe disease of all kinds. Maybe so. Maybe this malaria vaccine does a good job of generally cranking up the immune system, come what may. One wonders if this Gambia group consisted of all the children who were given the malaria vaccine. 100% prevention of malaria for 18 months in a place in sub-Saharan Africa seems too good to be true. Maybe they got lucky with a small sample size. On the other hand, they gave the vaccine to kids who were over 9 months old. So there wasn't any maternal antibodies to malarial antigens floating around to mess up the vaccines. 100% sterile protection for 18 months for kids over a year old sounds excellent.

The authors also cite a study from Mozambique where 65% of infants were protected from malaria by RTS,S/AS02D. The Mozambique group had malaria shots at different times than their other immunizations, staggered, say the authors, they also mention "a promising safety profile". That statement sounds good but it sounds like maybe some kids had bad reactions. It's probably too early to tell if any of them became autistic and how many. The authors don't mention what kind of preservative was used for the vaccines. I hope it's not thimerosal.

The authors gave the kids intramuscular shots in the left anterolateral thigh at 8, 12 and 16 weeks of age at the same time that other immunizations were given in the right thigh: diphtheria, tetanus, pertussis and flu all in one shot. That's not staggered, but it saves trips to the clinic. On the other hand, it might raise the possibility of a bad reaction. The vaccine seems to have helped keep around 60% of the kids from getting malaria for 7 months. The authors also mention that bed nets were distributed to families. This might have helped, but it's hard to tell how many used the nets. There's a lot of non-use of bed nets in Africa.

The authors say that low grade fever was reported in 29% of the kids after they got the malaria vaccine and the control kids didn't have this problem. The control kids got a hepatitis B vaccine. Sometimes you have to pay a price for whipping up the immune system. The authors mention that the children who got the malaria vaccine were less likely to get pneumonia than the control group, which might be due to the general immune system whip-up.

The authors say that about 25% of the kids had anti-sporozoite antibodies in their blood at the time of the first shot. The authors think the antibodies were received transplacentally before birth. I would guess that those anti-sporozoite antibodies would have reduced the effectiveness of the RTS,S, if not ruined it. On the other hand, maybe some kids had already had malaria. As we'll find later, there are parts of Africa where it's difficult to avoid it. This study makes RTS,S sound good. None of the children got very sick from the vaccine it seems. Hopefully none will become autistic. Break a bottle of wine on a tanker full of RTS,S and launch it. But wait! Maybe not so fast.

Here's an article that describes the results of a large study involving 15,460 children, some infants, phase 3 trials in 7 African countries. It seems the authors are convinced the vaccine works well. The authors say RTS,SAS01 can be safely administered with other childhood vaccines, but it turns out the RTS,S caused more convulsive seizures than the rabies vaccine within 7 days of the vaccine (9). That's a strong reaction. Rabies vaccines are known to cause seizures in dogs. Our cat never really recovered from a rabies vaccine he had, even though he lived another 5 years. He was violently ill for a couple days after the vaccination. If the RTS,S vaccine is causing more convulsions than rabies vaccines it sounds like a lot of convulsions. It's 18 seizures in the vaccinated group of 10,307 children. That doesn't sound like a lot, but "serious adverse events" occurred within 30 days of the vaccine in 1048 of 5949 older children, 17.6%. That sounds like a large percentage, but maybe some of them weren't caused by the vaccine. Hopefully there were no adverse events that cause brain damage or long-lasting neurological problems.

The authors say the children recovered from the seizures, but who knows what kind of brain problem they might have in the future? I would suggest not giving the malaria vaccine at the same time as other vaccines. In some cases it's too much stress on the immune system. Spread them out. And maybe the RTS,S vaccine needs to be made less toxic.

The authors say that 75% of the kids in their study used bed nets. This is a high percentage that no doubt helped many to survive. The authors say the vaccine reduced the likelihood of getting malaria by about half and if you got malaria you were only half as likely to get severe malaria. The authors also counted deaths, the rates of which were about the same in both experimental and control groups. The vast majority of deaths were not from malaria. The authors figure that so few died of malaria because they had access to high quality health care through the study. A lot of people using bed nets didn't hurt either. It's an encouraging study, but they should consider staggering the RTS,S vaccine with other vaccines rather than doing them all together in order to minimize the "serious adverse events". RTS,S will probably be approved but that's no reason to quit working on other malaria vaccines. RTS,S isn't perfect. Even despite having access to good health care and in some cases a malaria vaccine, some children in this study died of malaria.

The serious adverse events and seizures associated with RTS,S in this large study suggests to me that maybe they should try less toxic adjuvants. This would probably decrease the serious adverse events and seizures. It would do less to whip up the immune system and would probably result in less sterile immunity among those vaccinated, but you want to minimize the number infants and toddlers with bad reactions. My suggestion for RTS,S: use a milder adjuvant and rely on the malarial antigen to boost immunity to malaria. And maybe throw in another malarial antigen or two. You might not have as much sterile immunity, but it will still save lives and cut down on cases of severe malaria.

Another interesting thing about this study is that they had two age groups. One large group got their vaccines early, at 6-12 weeks of age. The other later, at 5-17 months of age. Vaccine "efficacy" was 55.8% for the older group and 34.8% for combined age categories. I don't why they didn't give the percentage for the younger group by itself. If the combined categories are young and old together, it seems the youngsters really dragged the percentage down. This might be explained by maternal anti-malarial antibodies that remove the vaccine from circulation before the immune system can process it. Maybe you should wait until 9 months of age, after maternal antibodies have cleared out, for malaria vaccines in Africa.

The authors of the next article look at a "family of parasite molecules", called Plasmodium falciparum erythrocyte membrane protein 1 (PfEMP1). It's actually a bunch of proteins coded by 60 or so genes that the parasite throws onto the surface of red blood cells after the parasite gets inside of it (10). These proteins mediate cyto-adhesion, which in malaria is a dangerous thing. When red blood cells stick to each other and the lining of blood vessels and whatever else, they can clog small vessels, which can result in human cells not receiving enough oxygen or nutrition to survive. This is the main way that malaria can kill you. So of course you're saying, "Hey! Let's zero in on these proteins for a vaccine." I agree. Blocking this protein, or a group of them, might not keep you from getting the disease, but it seems it might keep it from killing you.

The authors say, "Acquired immunity to Plasmodium falciparum infection causes a change from frequent, sometimes life-threatening, malaria in young children to asymptomatic, chronic infections in older children and adults." And they figure PfEMP1 is a key target of naturally acquired immunity. They cite another study that found that antibodies to infected erythrocyte surface molecules tend to protect children from clinical cases of malaria. So the kids might have merozoites in their blood cells and free-floating in their bloodstreams but not have any symptoms if they have the right antibodies.

The authors also mention that P. falciparum parasites are able to live in people for long periods without causing symptoms. They figure this might be a handy adaptation for keeping the parasites alive through the dry season, when there aren't as many mosquitoes around. The authors don't know why the human immune system doesn't wipe out the bugs sooner, but they suspect it has something to do with switching on and off genes in the PfEMP1 proteins. The immune system gets a bead on one set of proteins, but soon they're gone and another set pops up. Even so, the authors don't think PfEMP1 has enough genes to keep the infection chronic as long as it sometimes is. They speculate about how P. falciparum does it but don't say anything about a PfEMP1 vaccine. A bunch of antigens from this in a vaccine might keep the disease from becoming serious, or maybe even symptomatic.

This next article gives more details about the merozoite stage, and the antigens that might be used for a vaccine. They point out that parasite resistance to anti-malaria medicines is growing. They also mention that merozoites can develop inside red blood cells to form more merozoites (11). So you have merozoites coming from liver cells, but then more can come spurting out of red blood cells. Merozoites give rise to more merozoites. Maybe the idea is to really saturated your blood with them so that when a mosquito bites you it's for sure that she'll get some P. falciparum too.

The authors name merozoite surface proteins that help it enter both red and white blood cells, 6 for red and 3 for white that they specifically name, but there's more, probably all good targets for a vaccine that would probably lessen the symptoms of malaria and maybe prevent severe malaria.

Here's something that the authors say that I put a star beside, because it backs up my idea to get a malaria vaccine out SOON, even if it's not close to perfectly preventing the disease in all people: "Immunity to severe disease often develops before complete immunity is formed." Thank you very much dear authors! So if the vaccine doesn't completely prevent the disease in some people, there's a good chance that exposure to parasite antigens will give the vaccinated person additional resistance to the disease that they didn't have before, and result in less severe disease. Whoever is in charge of making malaria vaccines available to large numbers of people should have approved one long time ago. Expose young children's immune systems to malarial antigens to make the disease less severe when they get it. In some cases they may not get it at all. The idea of a single malaria vaccine for everyone might be less effective than a number of vaccines using different antigens at different stages of parasite development. Maybe with the right combination of vaccines people can expect to avoid the disease. But first you have to make some vaccines available. I say get them out there. The endless phases of trials are killing people.

The authors say that transfer of antibodies from immune donors to people with malaria results in reduced parasitemia and clears clinical symptoms. It's just a matter of getting the right antibodies, which, the authors say has not been figured out yet. Considering the many antigens of P. falciparum there are probably many different combinations that will clear the clinical symptoms. A different article states that adults in parts of Asia and Africa develop high levels of immunity to malaria but still harbor a low number of malaria parasites (12). Occasionally this gives rise to a "mild clinical state known as premonition", say the authors. One wonders why the immune system doesn't get rid of all the parasites. Maybe it's somehow disabled by the parasite or maybe the parasite has mechanisms for evading the immune system to some extent. If you've had a number of malarial infections over the years and the parasites have reached the sexual stage your small population of resident parasites might be evolving in response to your immune system and whatever drugs you use. P falciparum is a complicated group microbes with a lot of genetic diversity. If you move away from where you've lived for a long time in Africa to somewhere else in Africa, you can get a bad case of malaria because the local variety of P. falciparum is different from what your immune system is used to (4). To figure that you're going to get one vaccine that prevents malaria for a long time in almost all people seems overly optimistic. If you get a vaccine that can approximate that you might find that after a while some varieties of P. falciparum no longer have the antigens that the vaccine targets, due to evolution, especially if the vaccine only uses a small number of antigens.

The authors of the next article look at antibodies to malarial proteins in children from Papua New Guinea. They used 206 children and checked 46 proteins from the merozoite stage of P. falciparum. They found that new or understudied antigens were more associated with protection from malaria than the antigens used in current vaccine trials (13). They found that proteins used for parasite invasion of red blood cells are the ones especially targeted by immune systems that achieve high levels of protection. The authors also found combinations of antibodies that were strongly associated with protective immunity, where the antibodies by themselves didn't offer much protection. This might make sense if the proteins' functions were similar. If you disabled one the parasite can simply use the other one, but if you disable both, and there's no other way for the parasite to do that task, the parasite might be in trouble.

The authors say that merozoite antigen vaccines that have made it to phase 1 or 2 trials have showed "limited efficacy". Apparently there have been 6 antigens used in these trials. My guess is that if you get one of the vaccines of "limited efficacy" it might still help you to avoid severe malaria and death. Any head start your immune system has being better than nothing. But the authors seem to have found a way to evaluate antigens, in which case, let's try the high-value proteins, the ones that are apparently more important to the parasite.

You might think avoiding the disease would be the way to go, with bed nets, long sleeve shirts, screens on the windows. It might help, but the authors found that within 6 months 95.3% of their subjects were reinfected with P. falciparum. They got at least one more mosquito bite with malaria in it. The authors found this using PCR to identify the type of P. falciparum. 38% had an episode of symptomatic malaria. Maybe they should have said "at least one episode..." It's tough to avoid malaria in some parts of Africa.

The authors name 8 proteins known to be erythrocyte invasion ligands that they found to be associated with high levels of immunity when blocked. It seems the merozoite has more than one way to break in where it's not wanted. These ligands would probably be excellent targets for vaccines. Many antigen combinations showed additive effects, in other words, the more of them you include in a vaccine, the better, hopefully.

Even though the authors have done a terrific job of evaluating antigens for vaccines in a scientific way, they note that "almost all of the 46 antigens were associated with protection from symptomatic malaria at some level." The authors only looked at 46 antigens, and they were almost all associated with at least some protection. Get a bunch of those antigens and put them in a vaccine. If you can stifle the merozoites you can save lives, brains and other vital organs. Time's up on bullshitting around with this stuff. Make some vaccines available.

The authors say that many of the antigens they tested are not present in the rodent forms of malaria. So forget the preliminary mouse and rat studies. Finally, the authors give a list of 9 antigens of the 46 they studied that are associated with high levels of protection, which should be considered for vaccines. How about a vaccine with all 9? Sounds good to me.

The authors of the next article say there are doubts about the efficacy of any single or multi-antigen malaria vaccine, so they're pushing for a live vaccine with either radiation or genetic attenuation. Apparently they have a strict definition of "efficacy" because RTS,S seems pretty effective. It doesn't completely prevent malaria for everyone, or even close, but it does prevent it for a large fraction and also reduces severe malaria. That's some efficacy, and there are many more antigens and antigen combinations to try. Attenuated live vaccines are difficult to make and there are questions about how to administer them in a way easier than being bitten by 1000 mosquitoes.

The authors say that live attenuated vaccines established the benchmark for malaria vaccines by conferring "long lasting, sterile protection against infection (14)." Well, more recent live vaccine trials haven't performed so well. Nevertheless, the authors say that certain genetically engineered parasites give "complete sterile protection in animal malaria models", rodents, I'm guessing.

Live vaccines are preerythrocyte. The authors say that on the one hand, preerythrocyte stages show little genetic variation between different malaria strains, which makes for good vaccine targets that are present in most varieties of the sporozoite, while on the other hand, if even one sporozoite doesn't get killed, the person will probably get the disease. It seems the authors feel that the vaccine has failed if that one sporozoite survives. I would say that one surviving sporozoite might be a lot better than 50. If the one makes 10,000 merozoites the immune system has more time to adapt to the merozoites than if it is suddenly faced with 500,000 of them, which might result in a less severe disease and might even save a life. This idea that a malaria vaccine is a failure if it doesn't prevent the disease is wrong. The authors are confident that malaria can be eliminated with vaccines. I hope they're right, but it seems doubtful to me. In the meantime let's get some vaccines out there that fight the disease even if they don't eliminate it.

For radiation attenuated sporozoites, the authors note that a "precise irradiation dose" is required or the vaccine either won't work or it will give the person malaria. With subunit vaccines you don't have to worry about that. I would suggest, get a bunch of subunits on a vaccine, rather than just one. The authors also like the multi-antigen approach. They say that it's "conceivable that sterile protection can only be achieved by a multi-pronged immune response that targets many antigens." I agree. Make RTS,S available, but keep working on malaria vaccines. Better ones are on the way. Plus, it's possible that the parasites will evolve to lose antigens used by vaccines that are used a lot. In which case, it's time for a new vaccine.

The authors say that a company, Saravia Inc., has figured out a way to give sporozoites a precise dose of radiation and then to cryopreserve them. So you have to keep them cold. One wonders how precisely cold they have to be kept. It sounds like another way that the vaccine could be made useless. The authors say that >1000 infective mosquito bites with irradiated sporozoites confer sterile immunity for 10 months or more. Other methods of delivering the sporozoites haven't been nearly as good. When a mosquito bites you it probably injects some bacteria along with the radiation attenuated sporozoites. Maybe the bacteria along with the sporozoites does a better job of firing up the immune system. Maybe attenuated whole cell malaria vaccines need adjuvants too.

The authors say that whole cell vaccines in current trials are delivered by needle and syringe intradermally or sub-cutaneously. They say nothing about adjuvants. The authors say that radiation attenuated sporozoites have been found to persist alive in liver cells for up to 6 months. Maybe this gives the immune system time to zero in on a lot of antigens. And the fact that the parasite is alive might increase the immune response too. Maybe whole cell vaccines will be the way to go eventually, but they still need a lot of work, it seems, to reach their goal of near 100% sterile immunity. On the other hand, this kind of vaccine might give some degree of sterile immunity and reduce the chances for severe disease now, which means that it's not worthless. But if you've got subunit vaccines that can do the same thing, it's probably easier to go with the subunits.

The authors of the next article say, "blood-stage infection after sporozoite challenge is completely preventable by immunization with radiation attenuated sporozoites in mouse models of malaria (15)." They more or less say the same thing about genetically attenuated sporozoites. These authors are pushing for tests on humans for the genetically attenuated sporozoites they've been working on. The authors deleted a couple proteins in the parasite's vacuole, which it makes when it gets into a liver cell. Inside the vacuole it divides into 10,000 merozoites. Apparently nutrients can get through the vacuole wall to the 10,000 little beasts inside. By deleting the 2 proteins of the vacuole the development of the merozoites is stopped. Mice that got parasites with these deletions or the deletion of the P52 gene, were protected from mouse malaria. "Complete, long-lasting protection," say the authors, even with large numbers of wild type sporozoites injected. Unfortunately it's not going to do the world's mouse population much good.

The authors say that when you use single gene knockouts for the vaccine sometimes the vaccine will cause malaria rather than prevent it. You'll get a sporozoite or two that somehow reverts to the wild type. But when you knock out 2 genes that doesn't happen.

The authors mention that persistence in the liver cells was thought to be necessary to induce immunity by radiation attenuated sporozoites. But the authors say that's not true. Their genetically attenuated sporozoites apparently die quickly in the liver cells and they still induce lots of sterile immunity in mice. The authors are chompin' at the bit to do some human tests. They're gonna chomp their bits to bits. But they want to start their human studies by administering the vaccine through the bite of A. stephenski mosquitoes. One wonder how many bites will suffice for the vaccine, and how practical is it even if it does confer a high percentage of sterile immunity? I would suggest going straight for some kind of needle and syringe infection. While you're at it, try to figure out what kinds of bacteria and/or fungus are usually found on anopheles mosquitoes' mouths. Maybe you could throw in some of these microbes with the genetically attenuated parasite malaria vaccine, as an adjuvant.

The authors of the next study quote some World Health Organization figures that say that malaria kills up to 2.7 million people a year, mostly in Africa but also in Asia, Central America and South America (16). My brother sold a house in Mexico a while back. I looked at the pictures online and saw nets over all the beds, suggesting North America has some cases too. The authors say that people usually get immunity to malaria only "after several years of recurring infections and illness." What's more, this immunity is only partially effective. It doesn't keep you from getting the disease in all cases, but probably will result in milder symptoms. Then the authors say that even this degree of immunity is short-lived if not "reinforced by frequent reinfection." Even if they find a vaccine that prevents most cases of the disease, you might still need to have the vaccine or some malaria vaccine a number of times during your life if you live in the tropics in order to protect against severe malaria. The authors say that "in order to be effective a malaria vaccine must do better than the natural immune response." Once again it's the prevailing attitude among malaria researchers which unfortunately for the millions who die from malaria or get long-term neurological problems from it each year, is wrong. I'm sorry, but it's a stupid attitude. The human immune system generally does a good job of fighting malaria. Most people survive the disease and are OK neurologically afterward. If a vaccine is able to significantly reduce the number of symptomatic cases of malaria and the severity of the disease, that is a good vaccine. This idea that a vaccine has to be almost perfect is killing people, lots of them, while researchers receive more and more money from various governments and organizations in order to find "effective" vaccines. One might say the scientists are milking it, at the expense of people who actually get malaria. Maybe some of them worry that if people quit dying by the millions of malaria they'll be out of a job.

The authors say that it was the early 1970s when "a few human volunteers" were given multiple mosquito bites by irradiated mosquitoes carrying malaria sporozoites. The volunteers did not get malaria when bitten by mosquitoes with non-irradiated sporozoites. So, they irradiated the mosquitoes, that's how they irradiated sporozoites. The authors say that you can't just have a batch of sporozoites on hand. They don't survive in culture, but merozoites do. One wonders about the possibility of a live attenuated or dead merozoite vaccine. The authors seem to say that maintenance of any P. falciparum in culture is difficult, which reinforces the case for sub-unit vaccines. The authors mention a difficulty for sub-unit vaccines is that there are strain-specific antigens. In other words, you have different strains of P. falciparum with different antigens. That's a big problem with P. falciparum, it has lots of genetic possibilities. That's why a vaccine with multiple antigens might be the best way to go.

The authors say that even though blood-stage parasites are surrounded by "several membrane systems and develop within erythrocytes," some short peptides from that stage have been found to protect monkeys from P. falciparum blood stage disease. The blood stage is the symptomatic stage. To protect against this would be an excellent thing. It seems that if you get to where the merozoites are in your blood, the blood stage, even if you have a good vaccine for this stage you would probably have some disease symptoms, but if the symptoms are significantly reduced, you've got a winner.

The authors say that the first vaccine targeting blood stage antigens, SPF66, was tried in South American countries and resulted in a 39% reduction in clinical cases. The authors say that these numbers are encouraging enough to justify more attempts to improve efficacy. I say the numbers are encouraging enough to make the vaccine available now. The authors say the safety of the vaccine for adults and children has been established. Sure, continue working on it to make it better, but at the same time, make the present vaccine available. If it doesn't completely prevent the disease, chances are it will reduce the symptoms which is a hugely important goal. A vaccine aimed at the symptomatic stage of the disease would be expected to reduce the symptoms. The authors, with their warped sense of "efficacy" don't even mention the vaccines' effect on disease severity.

The authors do mention a number of other blood stage malaria antigens some of which have been found to induce immunity in animals. Maybe put a few in with the SPF66. The authors say that much of the mortality in malaria is due to "adherence of parasitized erythrocytes to the endothelium of cerebral and other capillaries." This is apparently true. The erythrocytes themselves can clump together too. The whole mess can lead to clogs in capillaries that supply brain cells, and other organs too. The authors say that ligands for this adherence have been difficult to identify. I see that this article was published in 1994, which suggests to me that a malaria vaccine should have been available to the public in the 1990s. At least some of the ligands that cause erythrocytes to become pathologically sticky have been identified in the 20 years since this was published. This is an old article, but it has some interesting stuff in it, and it was free.

The authors mention sexual stage malaria vaccines that wouldn't do the vaccinated person much good if they got bitten by a malaria-carrying mosquito, but it would help keep the disease from spreading. In some cases it would be too late to keep it from spreading because the person would be dead. A sexual stage vaccine is hardly worth mentioning. The authors didn't dwell on it either. Toward the end the authors say that an "effective" malaria vaccine appears to be coming along in the "near future". Well, it's 20 years later and still, nothing. But it's not because a truly effective vaccine hadn't been made and tested yet. It's because the egg-heads are holding out for perfection, even if it kills a million or so a year.

The authors of a more recent article say that malaria is "the leading cause of morbidity and mortality in sub-Saharan Africa despite tools currently available for its control (17)." Heart attacks, cancer, wars, they all fall in line after malaria, not necessarily in that order. Malaria is fucking up that whole continent. The authors mention some ways to fight malaria such as rapid diagnosis, prompt appropriate treatment, giving pregnant women sulphadoxine-pyramethamine intermittently, insecticide treated nets, and indoor bug spraying. I would suggest go easy on the sulpha drugs. My wife just had a bad reaction to Bactrim which caused us to have to sit in the ER for 2 hours during which they shot her up with steroids. The doctor said the reaction, which was a nasty rash quickly spreading to my wifes' throat and mouth, could have been much worse. Sometimes the rash can resemble third degree burns and has to be treated that way. On the other hand, I've taken Bactrim and never had a problem.

The authors mention that the bed nets get holes in them and are misused in other ways. I can picture a mosquito biting you through a net if the net was up against your skin. People with small houses or living spaces might not have the space to spread out a bed net the way it would work best, by never contacting skin. I would suggest getting good tight screens on windows to keep mosquitoes out at night. I've got screens on my bedroom window that look good, but if you open the glass on those windows in summer mosquitoes come in. I've found cracks around the edges of the screens not big at all, but big enough for a mosquito to get in. Mosquitoes are smart and determined.

The authors also mention that resistance to anti-malarial drugs is increasing. That's more or less a given. The parasites don't become less resistant. Artemisinin is the latest of the anti-malarial drugs. The authors say that resistance to it has been found along the Thia-Cambodian border. Hopefully it will continue to work well everywhere else for a while.

31

The authors say that the RTS,S vaccine is 30% and 50% effective in reducing cases of malaria in infants and children respectively even a year after vaccination. That's good for a vaccine that only targets one protein. My guess is that many if not most of the vaccinated kids who did get malaria during that year got less virulent cases. Even if it's not a perfect vaccine it's giving the immune system some kind of head start. After 4 years the RTS,S was only 16.8% effective in reducing cases of malaria, say the authors. It's still probably helping to reduce severe malaria in most kids by then, but it would probably be good to have an RTS,S booster sometime during the 4 years, or maybe better still, a different kind of malaria vaccine, like maybe SPF66. The little beasts have lots of antigens. Might as well take advantage of them.

The authors say that mosquitoes are becoming resistant to chemicals use to kill them. Plus, insecticides tend to kill the good insects too, like bees. Some of the older ones, like DDT, also killed animals, including humans. The newer insecticides are no doubt bad for humans too. We're not as different from mosquitoes as we think.

The authors say there are high rates of illiteracy in the part of Ghana where they did interviews and found that most people want their kids vaccinated against malaria as part of routine vaccinations. Education might be a big step toward reducing the effects of malaria in sub-Saharan Africa. My suggestion at least concerning the RTS,S vaccine, would be to not have it at the same time as other vaccines, since it potentially has some strong side effects, including seizures. The likelihood of this happening is increased when you give numbers of vaccines at once. Stagger them. It's a bit more inconvenient, but not as much so as having an autistic child. A dead child, you don't want that either. Give the youngster the best shot at a good life. You might also want to wait to give a malaria vaccine until 9 months of age. This would likely cut down on bad side effects and avoid having the vaccine inactivated by maternal anti-malarial antibodies. Up until then the child is protected by those antibodies for a while if the mother ever had malaria herself. If the kid is breastfed he or she will get non-specific anti-malarial protection from that. We'll get more into breastfeeding later.

The authors of the next article are excited about "Prime Boost" vectors for malaria vaccines. This means that you give a vaccine twice with a different vector each time, in this case, a DNA vector first and then with a modified vaccinia virus the second time a short while later. The authors say that when this was done there was a significantly lower number of parasites in the livers of those who got both of the different vaccines rather than two of the same vaccines (18). In all cases the vaccines contained TRAP, a liver-stage malaria antigen. In another test the authors say researchers used two different viral vectors with similar antigens, ME-TRAP, and reduced parasite burden in the liver by 90% after challenge by P. falciparum. 2 of 16 of the volunteers got sterile protection. The authors seem to say that the prime-boost formulation didn't work as well when given to 1-6 year-old children, 70% of whom showed "patent parasitemia". Just because you have patent parasitemia doesn't mean the vaccine is not working. It's probably still reducing the number of parasites you've got.

The TRAP antigen sounds like a good one for including in a malaria vaccine. It's already shown that it can work.. The authors say that in trials of TRAP with prime-boost vectors on Kenyan children the vaccines showed "no efficacy". Once again it seems that another group of authors use the word "efficacy" to mean complete prevention of the disease in those vaccinated. This is misleading because it makes it sound like the vaccines did the kids no good at all, when it probably reduced the severity of the disease in many if not all who got it. When you're talking about a disease that can kill you or leave you with brain damage, a vaccine that reduces the severity is effective. The more it reduces the symptoms the more effective it is.

The authors say that at least 25 malaria vaccines

have undergone "clinical efficacy testing" but only two have shown evidence of some "protective efficacy". I'm guessing that what they mean is that some of those vaccinated did not get the disease when challenged by P. falciparum. I also guess that the other 23 vaccines actually did offer some degree of protection but not enough to keep the disease from happening altogether. But probably enough to result in a less severe disease, which is an important goal, or should be. This article was published in 2010, so there's probably several more "clinical efficacy" tests to add to the list.

These same authors talk about vaccines that reduce parasite burden in liver cells by 80% and 90%. Even with the parasite burden reduced that much you'll still probably get malaria with symptoms, but my wild hunch is that it will be a milder disease than if you had to suffer through all 100% of your liver parasites.

The authors seem eager to see chimpanzee or simian viruses used as vectors for human vaccines. There's a possibility that HIV was originally a monkey virus of some sort that jumped to humans when they were making early polio vaccines. The whole idea of viral vectors does not sound great to me. The virus might "unexpectedly" revert to a pathological state. Also, many people already have some immunity to the viruses they want to use for vaccines, which might render the vaccine useless to them. The authors claim that some monkey viruses and human viruses are probably the same anyway. Maybe so, but the authors don't seem so sure.

The authors say that vaccines with the ME-TRAP antigens using a prime-boost strategy are still not good enough for deployment, even thought some people that have had them were protected from getting the disease at all. Most of the rest, if not all, were probably less likely to die of the disease or have long-lasting brain problems from it. I would say, if the vaccine is safe, doesn't cause sickness, it's a winner. Better still how about the ME-TRAP antigens without the prime boost, maybe combined with some other proven malaria antigens in a vaccine.

Once again, a group of serious researchers is ready to toss a good malaria vaccine in the garbage because it's not perfect. In the meantime people die.

The next group of authors write about merozoite surface protein 1 (MSP1), which is involved in red blood cell invasion. They say that in rodents and monkeys transfer of anti-MSP1 antibodies "can provide significant protection against lethal challenge (19)." It wasn't total protection, which is probably a disappointment to the authors, but the fact that some were protected shows that it works pretty well. Significant protection against lethal challenge is a great thing. If this translates to humans, even though it's not perfect, it's good. Even the best hitters in baseball mostly make outs. Just being able to get hits is something. These malaria vaccines maybe don't do everything you'd wish they would, but...

The authors say that some researchers have found that anti-MSP1 antibodies have enhanced parasitic growth. Of course other researchers have found just the opposite. You certainly don't want enhanced parasitic growth if you have malaria unless you're suicidal. If I didn't have several other major chores to attend to, including the replacement of the inner tie rod on our Grand Prix, I might track down those articles and try to find out who screwed up their experiment or its interpretation. OK, I'm lazy. The tie rod? I'm in no big rush to do that either. The authors seem convinced that MSP1 antibodies are good things to have if you live in places where malaria in found. They mention studies from New Guinea and Kenya where MSP1 antibodies were found a lot. In Kenya they correlated to the presence of immunity to malaria. In New Guinea those researchers consider MSP1 "a major component to the total inhibitory response." I suspect that an MSP1 vaccine would be good. Maybe a better approach would be to combine the MSP1 antigen with some other malaria antigens for more immune targets.

In case you were thinking that the attenuated sporozoite is the way to go for malaria vaccines, since it has produced sterile immunity in large percentages of those treated in some studies, the authors of the next article tell us that sporozoites cannot be raised in vitro. They have to be dissected out of mosquitoes salivary glands (20). You gotta have a steady hand for that. This article was written in 2008, which wasn't that long ago, but who knows? They might have figured out how to grow convenient piles of them by now, but I doubt it. The authors add that sporozoite vaccines need to be preserved at -140 degrees C. That's a hard temperature to maintain even in the Arctic. It seems that malaria vaccines for mass use will be made of sub-units for the near future.

The authors mention that one way that immunity to malaria can work is to have lots of antibodies "block sporozoite egress from the skin into the circulation and prevent invasion of target cells in the liver." The trick is to have enough anti-sporozoite antibodies in your blood to make that happen. If your antibodies only manage to block some of them, you're probably still better off than if all the sporozoites had their way. It might be the difference between life that death.

To further encourage fans of anti-sporozoite vaccines, the authors say that intravital microscopy has found that sporazoites stay at the site of the mosquito bite for several hours and some go to lymph nodes for a while, giving the immune system time to kill or cripple the sporozoites. It's not that much time, and if the immune system doesn't have some kind of previous exposure to the sporozoites, they'll probably get to the liver cells.

The authors say that a topical adjuvant might be a good way to whip up a stronger humoral response. They also consider the MSP1 antigen on the merozoite a good vaccine target. As long as there's a chance that some sporozoites will succeed in becoming tens of thousands of merozoites and causing symptomatic malaria, a malaria vaccine might as well target merozoites to some extent. The authors think that a malaria vaccine would do well to target all stages of the disease. I agree.

The authors of the next article, Noone et al., found that in the Nigerian villages where they worked 25% of the people had giant round worms, also known as Ascaris lumbricoides, which can grow to a foot long (21). Wikipedia says that 1/6 of the world's population is infected with them, mostly in tropical and subtropical places, more common where sanitation is not good or where they use raw human feces as fertilizer. They say Ascaris eggs are "one of the most difficult pathogens to kill." Bleach won't kill them, but cooking usually does. On their own, the eggs can survive 1-3 years.

Noone et al. Found that Ascaris lumbricoides infection had no impact on P. falciparum parasitemia or immune responses to malaria. Nevertheless, they say that A. lumbricoides infection can be protective against severe forms of P falciparum. One of the studies they cite for this, M. Nacher et al., speculate that the worm infection might decrease cyto-adherence, which would possibly reduce the clogging of capillaries and other blood vessels in the brain caused by cerebral malaria. Maybe so. But maybe the worm infection has a stimulating effect on the immune system in a non-specific way that helps it fight P. falciparum. The BCG vaccine has been found to protect to some extent against malaria and doesn't contain malaria antigens. We'll get to more about that later. It seem that challenges to the immune system in general can sometimes make the immune system stronger against pathogens in general.

Noone et al. Suggest that a strong immune response might actually cause malaria symptoms, especially cerebral malaria, to be worse. They say that cerebral malaria is most common in kids 2-4 years old. They say a strong immune response to malaria is good and helps clear out the parasites, but "if these robust inflammatory responses are not tightly regulated, they can lead to immunopathology and severe forms of malaria." So it seems from this that the immune system could use some help. Rather than having a billion merozoites to deal with, a few million might be easier to handle without the immune system overreacting and causing "immunopathology". This might be accomplished by giving the person a vaccine that targets sporozoites. Even if it didn't kill all of them, reducing their numbers would probably reduce the danger of immunopathology.

On the other hand, a vaccine that targets merozoites would probably make it easier for the immune system to fight them and get rid of them, making it less likely that the immune system will become overactive and somehow cause cerebral malaria. I say get a vaccine that targets both sporozoites and merozoites. In some cases it might give people sterile protection for a while and the rest will probably get some protection against severe malaria.

I'm not sure if I should bother including this next article. The authors say that the removal of circulating immune complexes is necessary in malaria to avoid over-stimulation of the immune system (22). Immune complexes in this case are malaria pathogens or parts of them with antibodies and or complement stuck to them to make the parasites non-functional and label them for destruction. Unfortunately you can have a lot of these in your blood if you have malaria. CR1 receptors on a number of immune cells help to get rid of immune complexes, but the authors say CR1 receptors are down-regulated during malaria infections. What might seem like an odd coincidence is that human red blood cells also have CR1 receptors, which is one of the ways malaria parasites use to enter them.

CR1 receptors also cause red blood cells to attach to one another say the authors, which contributes to rosetting, which is when a bunch of them stick together. Rosetting has been linked to cerebral malaria. Maybe the immune system puts out a general order to down-regulate CR1 receptors to make it harder for malaria parasites to get into red blood cells. But then you're stuck with more immune complexes floating around, causing trouble.

Just when you think it all makes sense, the authors tell you that another immune trigger, LPS, lipopolysacharide, also caused CR1 receptors to be down-regulated. They don't say how much it was down-regulated or how much LPS they used. Maybe there's a mechanism to avoid burning out all your immune cells when you suddenly have a huge amount of garbage in your blood.

My idea for dealing with the sudden massive pile of crap in your blood that happens with malaria is to use a vaccine to give the immune system a head start. Even if you don't completely prevent the disease, a vaccine can help lessen the severity of it. We've wasted enough time waiting for the perfect malaria vaccine. Time to settle for something less in order to save lives and brains of some people, even if they do get the disease. The authors also mention that the CR1 receptor is down-regulated in both P. falciparum and P. Vivax types of malaria. P. Vivax malaria is rarely fatal. It's not nearly the killer P. falciparum is. It's interesting what the authors found out about the CR1 receptor but it doesn't seem to be the key to P. falciparum's deadliness, unless it's a matter of degree. Maybe P. falciparum is able to down-regulate CR1 a lot more than P. Vivax or most other inflammatory stimuli. If that's the case I would suggest that it might be P. falciparum's ability to throw such a huge amount of garbage into your blood very quickly that makes it such a powerful CR1 down-regulator. A vaccine to get rid of some sporozoites before they become 10,000 merozoites each, and more as the merozoites invade red blood cells and make more merozoites, might reduce P. falciparum's ability to down-regulate CR1 receptors, which should result in a milder disease.

The next article is titled "Immunological disturbances associated with malarial infection". The authors say that malarial parasites are able to hinder antibody production, avoid antigen recognition, and keep infected cells alive (23). The authors say that intact red blood cells have been seen with "degenerating parasites" inside. Normally you'd figure the immune system would get rid of that whole red blood cell.

Here's an item from this article that's not encouraging: they say immunity to malaria is "strain specific". I've seen this before, that people get more or less immune to the malaria in their area, but then they get malaria again if they move somewhere not too close. If you move to somewhere where malaria is not endemic and stay there for a while, the authors don't say how long, you'll lose your immunity to malaria. What this suggests to me is that if you expect to find one malaria vaccine that will prevent the disease for life, quit dreaming. These little monsters can throw too many antigens at you and have devious ways of manipulating the immune system. But that doesn't mean you can't fight them with vaccines. They have lots of antigens to chose from. I suspect that with a combination of antigens we can make malaria vaccines that dramatically reduce the death toll and number of neurologically impaired from malaria.

Maybe a vaccine with one antigen, such as RTS,S could do this. But malaria vaccines might only be truly effective for a while before P falciparum evolves ways to defeat it. The authors mention P. falciparum's "ability to alter its surface molecules through various maturational stages." You'd think that after a bout or two of malaria you'd be immune, but it apparently takes more than that. It's a tough bug for the immune system to focus on. The authors also mention the delicate equilibrium between effective immunity and disease-inducing immunopathology." That can happen during the blood stage when the immune system is suddenly faced with large numbers of merozoites. If the immune system can kill some sporozoites before they get to the liver or any other cell and become 10,000 merozoites each and if the immune system can recognize and kill a large number of the first wave of merozoites, my guess is that you won't have to worry as much about immunopathology. That's probably more likely with an immune system that doesn't recognize the parasites until there's already a super huge number of them in your blood. A vaccine might make the difference between a huge number of parasites and a super-huge number, which might be the difference between life and death.

The authors say that "early innate immune response to malarial infection is important for controlling parasite growth." This is probably why the BCG vaccine, which contains no malarial antigens, gives some degree of protection against malaria. It's a tuberculosis vaccine, but apparently it whips the whole immune system in shape, including the innate part, the part that is non-specific. If that part of your immune system is thoroughly ready for action your chances are better if you are unfortunate enough to get malaria.

The authors say "Studies on malarial infection during pregnancy report a general decline in immunity which puts the mother and fetus at increased risk of death." A pregnant woman's immune system is constantly exposed to fetal antigens. Maybe the maternal immune system has to be dialed down to some extent during pregnancy in order for the child to survive, which gives malarial parasites more opportunities to proliferate. Generally speaking, the more parasites that escape the immune system, the worse the prognosis, I'm guessing. Although there are people who can have fairly high levels of parasitemia and do not have many if any symptoms. This makes one suspect that at least some of the symptoms of the disease are due to immune reaction to it. My suggestion is to keep parasite burden as low as possible by helping the immune system to kill off a lot of them early so they can't multiply.

The authors of this article say that circulating immune complexes are rarely found in uncomplicated cases of malaria. That earlier article we looked at seemed to say that circulating immune complexes (CICs) are found in malaria in general. If some malaria cases don't have CICs then it could mean that some strains of malaria have some kind of mechanism for disabling the immune system to some degree that other strains don't have. On the other hand, maybe the uncomplicated cases are those where parasite burden is lower and doesn't overwhelm the immune system so much that it can't process all the immune complexes. But then, like I said before, some people seem to be able to handle fairly high levels of parasitemia with few symptoms. Maybe those are more benign strains or maybe their immune systems have come to tolerate the parasites to a large extent.

The immune system with regard to malaria is still quite a mystery, at least to me. Those that can tolerate high parasitemia levels are generally those who have had a bunch of cases of the disease, and are at lower risk of dying from malaria. They've probably made the cut already, in terms of life and death. But they might have lost some brain cells in the process. Even a malaria vaccine that is not perfect and doesn't prevent the disease in almost all cases, which maybe only prevents the disease in relatively few cases, should be expected to significantly lower death rates and rates of serious brain injury, because you're giving the immune system a head start.

Rosetting

This section is about rosetting of malarial red blood cells, which causes them to stick together, sometimes in bunches, in which condition they can clog small blood vessels. If enough blood vessels in the brain get clogged, you know what happens. I won't even say the word because it's so grim. OK, OK, I'll say it: death. I started to try to put the articles in this section in some kind of sensible order, but I've given up on that, so we might jump around a bit, but I hope not.

The authors of the first article in this section say that a couple different thalassemias and the sickle cell trait, which are genetic variations in the formation of red blood cells, confer some protection against death and severe disease due to malaria (24). The authors find that this is probably due to reduced rosette formation. The authors say that kids with the sickle cell trait have 90% protection against cerebral malaria. That sounds great. Unfortunately kids with sickle cell disease, who get the trait from both parents, are more likely to have severe malaria than those without the trait at all.

In case you doubt that rosetting is such a bad thing, the authors say that "Increased frequency of spontaneous erythrocyte rosetting around parasitized red blood cells has been shown to be associated with cerebral malaria at autopsy." In ex-vivo experiments blood flow obstruction was "considerably more pronounced" when rosetting took place, say the authors. Here's something even more pertinent in this article, children with milder malaria were frequently found to have anti-rosetting antibodies in their blood, while those with severe disease had little or none of them. Hey, how about a vaccine aimed at producing anti-rosetting antibodies? If they can recognize these antibodies it seems they ought to be able to use a vaccine to produce them.

The authors say low red blood cell volume, which is characteristic of thalassemias, which give some protection against malaria, are associated with reduced ability of the small cells to form rosettes. The authors say that microcytosis of any kind, genetic or otherwise, hinders rosette formation. You can't make a vaccine that reduces blood cell size, but it's evidence that rosetting is a deadly feature of malaria. The authors say that other characteristics of tiny blood cells have been investigated and found not to have any hindering effect on malaria. The authors also say that yes, rosetting is inhibited by sickled blood cells too. Even so, it seems that if you have full bore sickle disease you're at much worse risk of death from malaria if you get it. Maybe even the little rosetting that happens to sickle cell sufferers when they get malaria is enough to push your already screwed up blood off the cliff, and you with it.

The authors say that rosette formation is mediated by protein ligands called rosettins on infected red blood cells that latch onto carbohydrate receptors on uninfected red blood cells. How about a vaccine that targets rosettins? The authors say that these ligands and receptors are found on the red blood cells of those with the sickle cell trait and those with the disease, but the shape of the cells tends to keep them from linking up as much. Since the sickle cell

43

trait is the best known of a bunch of genetic mutations thought to have spread in the world as a result of malaria, it suggests that the aspect of the disease that it affects, rosetting, is the most deadly of malaria's symptoms, and an excellent target for a vaccine.

The authors of the next article point out that genetic red blood cell disorders are almost all found in malaria endemic regions (25). They mention thalassemias, sickle cell trait, and hemoglobin C, which also confers protection against malaria. The authors say it does this through an abnormal display of the malarial antigen PfEMP1 on the surface of red blood cells, which reduces cytoadhesion and rosetting, giving the carriers of this mutation a much better chance of surviving malaria and not becoming permanently messed up doing it. How about a vaccine with PfEMP1 in it? A large batch of antibodies to this protein might significantly reduce rosetting, saving lives and keeping brains functioning well. A vaccine consisting of PfEMP1 as the only malarial antigen would be unlikely to prevent cases of malaria, but it would stand an excellent chance of reducing the most deadly symptoms, cytoadhesion and rosetting.

Rowe et al., the authors of the next article, talk about 3 different kinds of adhesion problems of parasitized red blood cells in malaria: binding to endothelial cells (on the inside lining of blood vessels), rosetting with uninfected red blood cells, and platelet-mediated clumping of red blood cells (26). This article goes into detail about aspects of red blood cell adhesion problems with malaria. They say in 1-2% of cases life-threatening disease develops. You know it's bad when these things happen: impaired consciousness, coma, difficulty breathing, severe anemia, and multi-organ failure. The authors say the problems are thought to be caused by high parasite burden and sequestration of infected red blood cells in microvascular beds throughout the body. The authors add that sequestration helps the parasites because it keeps the red blood cells they live in away from the spleen, which would remove and destroy them.

The authors point out differences in low and high transmission areas of the world. They say that in southeast Asia, a low transmission area, severe malaria hits all ages. But in sub-Saharan Africa, where transmission is high, severe disease is usually found in children under 5. It all has to do with immunity through previous exposure to the disease. In southeast Asia a person can go years or even decades without getting malaria, but probably not in sub-Saharan Africa. You'll see later that in Africa you can get malaria on top of malaria during high transmission season. That's gotta be bad, unless the first type of malaria is Plasmodium vivax, which seems able to induce some immunity to P. falciparum, which we'll get to later also.

The authors, Rowe et al., say there's a direct link between total parasite burden and disease severity and death in southeast Asia. But in Africa they say some children tolerate "extremely high parasitemia" without major problems. Maybe these kids have immune systems that make antibodies that inhibit rosetting and/or other forms of malaria-induced red blood cell adhesion.

Some of the previous authors suggested that disruption of rosetting might raise parasitemia which they thought might have dangerous effects. Maybe people can handle lots of malaria parasites in their blood if they don't form rosettes and block small blood vessels. Rowe et al. say that in Africa severity of disease in children is associated with rosetting. My guess is that in southeast Asia if you die of P. falciparum malaria, there' probably some rosetting and other forms of red blood cell adhesion that gummed things up.

The authors say that the parasite protein PfEMP1 is "responsible for at least some of the adhesive properties of IEs (infected erythrocytes)," which suggests to me that maybe PfEMP1 is responsible for all of them. The authors don't seem to know of any other parasite proteins that cause erythrocyte adhesion. So you might think, "OK, lets get a vaccine with PfEMP1 and we should be right in line for the Nobel prize. Well, the authors also point out that P falciparum has about 60 genes for this protein and it can switch these genes often. So you might have a good vaccine for one PfEMP1, but not all the other possible varieties. On the other hand, it occurs to me that there are probably some parts of PfEMP1 that are the same, or close to it, as most other PfEMP1s. Maybe go for those parts of the protein, or several of the more common PfEMP1s in a vaccine. If you can eliminate rosetting from malaria, go ahead and start writing your speech, start looking at tuxes, check craigslist for a nice used Porche.

Rowe and associates say that it was known as early as the 1890s that red blood cells would bind to endothelial cells in small blood vessels in some cases of malaria, which was found by autopsies. They add that there's a bunch of receptors P. falciparum can use to do this, the best studied being CD36 and ICAM1. The authors say that even though CD36 is found on many types of human cells, including endothelial cells, macrophages, monocytes, platelets, and erythrocyte precursors, they don't seem to have a major role in severe malaria. But who knows? The authors say that when the parasite links to dendritic cells through CD36 it inhibits the immune response of those cells and causes dendritic cell precursors not to mature. Messing with the human immune system seems to be one of the major effects of malaria.

When infected red blood cells bind to ICAM1 they use PfEMP1, but only some varieties of PfEMP1 have the ICAM1 binding ability, so it seems this receptor also does not play a major role in severe malaria, say the authors. It would be nice to know what the main receptor in the human body is for severe malaria because maybe you could block it, although it seems the parasite is able to use a number of different receptors.

From the perspective of the vaccine maker you'd want to figure out ways to block the most likely parts of PfEMP1 to link up with endothelial cells and red blood cells. The authors say that CD36 binding can be done by almost all varieties of P. falciparum. If you could discover the parts of PfEMP1 that bind to CD36 those parts might be good for a vaccine. But the authors tell about 6 other receptors that P. falciparum binds to, and they mention a bunch more possible receptors after that.

PfEMP1 seems like sort of a skeleton key in more ways than one, since it can also make you into a skeleton pretty quickly. When endothelial cells in blood vessels get latched onto by infected red blood cells it can cause the endothelial cells to malfunction. They might undergo apoptosis (programmed cell death) or they might lose the ability to dilate their blood vessel, say the authors, who add that this is due to low nitric oxide (NO) levels. Blood vessels dilate in response to lack of oxygen to get more oxygen carrying blood in. What's more, the authors say that NO tends to prevent adhesion by down-regulating adherence receptors.

The authors say that the force of blood flow usually keeps rosettes from happening on the arterial side. It's the postcapillary venules, where blood is moving slow, where the adhesion and clogging happen.

When it comes to ways for PfEMP1 to link up with red blood cells, the authors say there are generally three receptors on the red blood cell that are used: CR1, heparin-sulphate-like molecules, and the A or B blood group antigens. But they add that good ol' CD36 is also on erythrocytes in small numbers. The A blood group antigens seem to be the worst, according to this article. If you're type O you're at reduced risk of dying of malaria, since type O is the absence of A and/or B antigens. I'm type A. I'll just look at pictures of Africa, thank you. Have a nice trip.

The authors add that some antibodies might also contribute to rosetting. I suppose so, since the antibodies can be there in the small vessels taking up space too. But if you can get antibodies that reduce adhesion of blood cells and endothelial cells it seems logical that the antibodies would help keep blood flowing normally. On the other hand, antibodies that are induced by other malarial antigens might in some cases help to clog things up. Hopefully this tendency would be counteracted by the antibodies' ability to eliminate parasites.

The authors say that the part of PfEMP1 that binds to CR1 is known. This would probably be a good target for a vaccine. The part of PfEMP1 that binds to the blood group A antigen has been discovered, say the authors. It's not a great vaccine possibility since it wouldn't do anyone with types B or O blood any good. But it's good practice.

The authors say that if you get severe malaria there's a 15-20% chance that you'll die. They say people who come to the hospital with severe malaria, even well-equipped hospitals, often die, usually within the first 24 hours, too early for standard antimalarials to have any effects, which the authors say can take up to 24 hours. The authors say that artemesinin drugs kill malaria parasites at all stages of their development, unlike quinine, which doesn't. They might add that these drugs work if the strain of malaria is not resistant to them. As more and more people use antimalarial drugs the parasites will become more resistant to them. There's not a wide range of drugs for killing P. falciparum, but the parasites have a huge range of proteins and antigens to explore for vaccine targets. Let's make the vaccines available and keep new ones coming.

The authors say that you can raise a person's NO levels by giving them intravenous L-argenine, which can be made into NO easily by the human body. They say NO has anti-adhesive effects and L-argenine improves endothelial function in adults with moderately severe malaria, however that is defined.

The authors say that heparin can reverse rosetting in 30%-50% of cases, which limits its usefulness. Yes, I suppose it does limit it some. I wonder how often kids with severe malaria in Africa are given heparin. I'll bet not too often. The authors say that curdlan sulphate has "broader rosette disrupting activity" and that soluble CR1 receptors given to patients also have some anti-rosetting activity. Between the three of those you probably have quite a bit of anti-rosetting but you would have to get to a well-equipped hospital or clinic to get them. Nevertheless, you could probably save some lives.

The authors mention that aspirin reverses platelet binding, which might get blood flowing a bit better for those with severe malaria, but they add that platelets are also important parasite killers. So if you want to keep blood flowing it's probably best to think of ways other than disabling platelets.

How about this statement by the authors as one that PETA might quote: "None of the primate or rodent models develop clinical and pathological features similar to those in humans." What they're talking about is severe malaria in humans. It's time to end animal experimentation. It's torture and murder of innocent animals that just want to have a decent life, the same as you and me. Be creative. Think of non-cruel ways to do experiments. I suppose it sounds hypocritical of me to say this while at the same time I quote studies that feature experiments on animals. But I'm not supporting them financially in any way. I get all these articles for nothing. Even so, having a highly renowned biological writer such as me quote your article is surely some kind of ego and/or career boost, which the torturers shouldn't get. Sorry about that.

While we're on the subject, go vegan. Seriously, make yourself healthier and give animals a better chance at a good life. You'll feel better in every way, but don't forget to take some vitamin B-12 every now and then. Here's my suggestion for taking vitamin B-12: break up the pill into small pieces. If you take the whole thing you might get a headache. The pills I have are 500 micrograms, which is 8333% of the minimum daily requirement. I took 2 of them a couple weeks ago and had a terrible headache the next day. When I looked it up online other people had similar experiences.

Back to this malaria article. The authors end by saying that for many people who make it to the hospital with severe malaria it's too late. They die. For these people, a vaccine or two might have saved their lives, vaccines that have already been tested on humans. With P. falicparum's huge range of antigens and stages, there are

49

many possibilities for effective vaccines that save lives and prevent malaria from becoming severe.

The authors, Tembo et al., of this next article say that the placenta is "a site of preferential pRBC (parasitized red blood cell) accumulation (27)." I would guess that this results in many stillbirths caused by malaria. The authors figure they know the main receptor in the placenta for the adhesion, chondroitin sulphate A. The authors cite some studies that apparently show that CD35 is a receptor associated with rosetting and severe disease. Our previous authors who mentioned quite a few receptors that the little beasts can use to cause problems, didn't mention this one. Maybe the parasites can grab onto almost anything sticking out a little. I hope that's not the case.

Here's another human receptor that Tembo et al. say can cause pRBC to stick to things: gClgR/HABf1/p32. The authors think this receptor may have accounted for the accumulation of platelets found in the brain microvasculature of Malawaian children who had died of malaria. Maybe for these kids some disabling of platelets by a drug like aspirin would have helped them keep the microvessels clear. Maybe it's a matter of timing when it comes to giving aspirin to people with malaria. Maybe you only give it to them in cases of cerebral malaria, to keep brain vessels unclogged at the price of letting some parasites escape destruction by the immune system. Apparently cerebral malaria can use up lots of platelets, many of which get trapped in microvessels.

The authors say that the thrombocytopenia found in people with cerebral malaria is enough to "limit the further formation of pRBC clumps in vitro." This suggests that platelets have a role in malaria-caused blood cell clumping and adhesion. If aspirin really could help people with severe and/or cerebral malaria it would be terrific, since it's cheap and available. But once again, taken at the wrong time it might make the disease worse. By the time a person has cerebral malaria it might be too late to expect them to swallow aspirin pills. They might need intravenous aspirin. In that case they need a trip to the hospital or clinic that hopefully has the equipment and staff that know what to do. On the other hand, if the person had had a malaria vaccine, the disease might never have become that serious.

This next article that I will be forcing into your eyeballs contains an amazing statistic. The authors say that in Mali, which is in Africa, during the peak malaria transmission months, which are July to December, a person can expect 20-60 malaria infected mosquito bites per month (28). That really makes it seem like forget it, you're not going to avoid this crap.

Maybe cutting down on the number of infective bites would lessen the severity of the disease. Most children in Mali at that time of year probably suffer to some degree from overlapping cases of malaria, possibly with different strains of the disease at the same time. I just checked out the architecture of villages in Mali. It looks like mostly mud huts where the mud bricks have to be replaced every year after the rainy season. The pictures I saw on the internet of the houses, which are very small, don't show any screens on the windows. There are surely advantages to mud huts. They're cheap. It's not hard to find mud. Maybe they even keep you kind of cool in the night. But having houses with screens on the doors and windows would almost surely cut down on malaria transmission. This would require money. In the short term malaria vaccines might be a more practical way to keep people from dying of malaria.

The authors mention patients with hyperparasitemia, which they say is greater than 500,000 parasites per micro liter of blood. They add that some people that have this have no other signs or symptoms of disease. A micro liter is way under a teaspoon. It's a tiny amount of liquid. That means these people with hyperparasitemia have literally gazillions of parasites in them. These people either have strong well-adapted immune systems and/or less virulent strains of malaria. The researchers in this article were concerned about clumping of red blood cells, which they consider different from rosetting.

Despite what the authors say about asymptomatic people with huge parasite loads, they found that children with uncomplicated malaria had lower parasitemia levels. Of 51 children with severe malaria the authors assessed, 16 had unrousable coma, 12 non-comatose had impaired consciousness or prostration (defined online as complete physical or mental exhaustion), 14 with repeated seizures, 5 with severe anemia, and 4 others with jaundice, hematuria, and renal failure. Those are all very discouraging symptoms. If you have a young child with these things happening it's got to be a heart-breaker. 18 of these kids had hyperparasitemia. It seems logical that hyperparasitema in children is often accompanied by severe symptoms.

The authors say that clumping was strongly associated with parasitemia, which seems logical. But then they say clumping is negatively associated with rosetting. For me this is unexpected. Maybe the immune system can gauge the overall adhesiveness of blood, so when the rosettes appear the immune system reduces clumping by reducing platelets or deactivating them. The immune system might do this to avoid clogged blood vessels. The authors mention that platelets are known to inhibit the growth of parasitized red blood cells,

They say that rosetting might be a way for the parasites to avoid the immune system by reducing the number of platelets. This might promote hyperparasitemia which would be a benefit to the parasites. If a hyperparasitized person is bitten by a mosquito it's likely the mosquito will pick up a lot of parasites. In the authors' study rosetting frequency was strongly associated with severe disease, during which you can picture the sufferer in many cases being too incapacitated to be able to swat a mosquito. While they're laying there close to death they're easy sources of blood for mosquitoes, blood that is loaded with P. falciparum.

The authors found that clumping is not associated

with high parasitemia. This might be because clumping is part of an effective immune response. The authors say that, "Non-severe hyperparasitemia is a feature of malaria in children in semi-immune populations such as those found in sub-Saharan Africa." Semi-immune means that these people have some resistance to malaria already, probably because they've had it at least once before. They're not completely immune, because they can still get the disease, but their semi-immunity keeps them from suffering severe symptoms. This semi-immunity might include antibodies to parts of PfEMP1 that help form rosettes. Semi-immunity like this is probably achievable now with vaccines. A vaccine that includes anti-rosetting antigens would surely save lives. The authors say that rosetting takes place via PfEMP1. Latching some antibodies on to that might be a major jackpot winner.

The authors of the next article, Leitgeb et al., say that heparin has been used to treat severe malaria but it caused major bleeding in at least one case so they quit using it (29). Sounds like they gave someone or some people too much of it. The authors say that heparan sulphate is a receptor on red blood cells that is involved in rosetting, and that heparin does help disrupt rosettes and in some cases improves malaria symptoms.

The authors say that researchers have found a part of PfEMP1, the molecule that malaria parasites put on the outside of red blood cells that makes the RBC form rosettes, that binds to heparan sulphate. This little chunk they call DBL1α. When they immunized rats and monkeys with DBL1α. The animals showed less sequestration of parasitized red blood cells. A vaccine with DBL1α for humans might save lives. If you can cut down on rosettes the disease will almost surely be less severe. DBL1α sounds like a good candidate antigen for a vaccine.

The authors say that both heparin and heparan sulphate bind directly to DBL1α of PfEMP1. So heparin blocks that part of the parasite rosette connector. Good riddance to that. The authors say when heparin was used in the past it caused intracranial bleeding in some cases, but now, the low anticoagulant heparin won't do that, or is less likely to. That's great. But there are people who won't ever get to the hospital to get heparin. For them, a vaccine that blocks rosette linkages would be better. I'm no expert on Africa but my impression is that there are many people there without ready access to a good hospital.

The authors say that other receptors on red blood cells that are used in rosetting are the A blood group antigen and the CR1 receptor. If you figure out what the ligands for these are on parasitized red blood cells they might be good vaccine candidates too. Of course a vaccine aimed at the A blood group antigen won't help everybody. Monika Gandhi says that blood group B antigens can also act as receptors for resetting. She mentions other receptors involved in rosetting: ICAM-1, thrombospondin, E-selectin, chondroitin sulphate, CR1, and CD36. It seems the parasites have quite a few options (30). Even so, she figures that CR1 plays "a very important role in malaria pathogenesis." Tham et al. say that CR1 is also involved in letting malaria parasites into red blood cells (31). They have even found the parasite ligand involved. That ligand in a vaccine might be helpful. If you could block CR1 binding to PfEMP1 with a vaccine you'd probably save lives, and cutting down on entrances by the parasite into the RBC would be an added plus.

Leitgeb et al. say that not only might low anticoagulant heparin (LAH) be useful for disrupting rosettes, but that it inhibits merozoite invasion of red blood cells in vitro. P. falciparum really knows its way around the human red blood cell. The authors say that LAH was safe to use, showed no severe adverse effects, and was well tolerated in phase I trials. That's great, but you still have to get to a hospital or clinic to use it unless you can get someone to make a house call.

Leitgeb et al. say that another group found that in Gambia 30% of people given heparin had greater than 50% disruption in rosettes. Even a 20% disruption in rosettes might save lives. Leitgeb et al. say that LAH also disrupts cytoadherence, which would include blood vessels. It sounds like LAH is a good treatment for severe malaria if you can get it to the people who need it. On the other hand, a vaccine that targets the parasite ligands that interact with heparan sulphate on red blood cells might keep people from becoming severely ill in the first place. It sounds like they've already figured out what one of those ligands on PfEMP1 is, DBL1α. Include it in a vaccine and keep looking for more ligands.

The authors of the next article, Juillerat et al. say that heparin and other sulfated oligosacharides can disrupt rosettes (32). Maybe everyone in Africa should be given a big syringe full of heparin or some other sulfated oligosacharide every so often, just in case. The authors found that for the variety of malaria they tested heparin inhibited rosettes in a dose-dependent way. Of course we've learned from the previous article that too much heparin can cause bleeding in your brain, which is bad. Maybe hold off on those free syringes for everyone.

Juillerat et al. say that PfEMP adhesins expressed on the surface of infected red blood cells "are clustered in knob-like structures" that can interact with "diverse host receptors". You'd like to get a mini scissors and cut all those knobs off. Juillerat et al. say that for a variety of receptors rosetting is inhibited by heparin. These authors never mention bleeding problems. Maybe you just have to be careful not to give a person too much. Maybe there are different concentrations of heparin that are easy to confuse with one another. The authors caution that heparin may enhance adhesion of parasitized red blood cells to microvascular endothelium. They cite a study for this which I didn't look up. Sorry. Maybe heparin leaves more infected RBCs floating around because fewer are in rosettes so this results in more infected RBCs being available to stick to blood vessel walls. So it looks like heparin is not perfect. Nevertheless, if it can inhibit a lot of rosettes and only slightly increase adhesion to blood vessel endothelium, it would probably save lives.

The authors say that rosette stability ranges from loose to tight depending on the receptors used. It might be difficult for a vaccine to duplicate heparin's multiple receptor anti-rosetting activity. But if a vaccine made a few of those receptors unusable by PfEMP1 that might be enough to save a significant number of lives of children who wouldn't get to the hospital in time.

This next article says that a vaccine to prevent severe malaria is a realistic goal. It seems the authors have found a way to inhibit rosetting in at least some cases. They start off by saying that vaccines against PfEMP1, the malaria adhesion molecule, have had problems due to "extensive sequence diversity (33)". They say that PfEMP1s from different parts of the world show "essentially unlimited amino acid sequence diversity", which sounds discouraging, like the parasite's got all the aces.

But the authors also note that children in endemic areas generally become immune to severe malaria in the first few years of life. I would add, if it doesn't kill them first. The authors reason that strain transcending antibodies are probably acquired by that early age with relatively few infections. This is why vaccines could probably reduce severe disease, or maybe eliminate it, by inducing the strain transcending antibodies. The authors say their induction of strain-transcending antibodies to PfEMP1 variants implicated in severe childhood malaria is the first of its kind that they know of. These authors are looking at the same region of PfEMP1 that Lietgeb et al. mention, NTS-DBLα, although they use a few other letters from the Greek alphabet also. If it turns out that these antigens only give immunity to severe disease to a smaller than hoped for number of cases, don't toss it out. Keep it. It's a start. For a parasite with such a huge number of possible antigens you might need to include quite a few of them from different varieties of parasites to get one or two vaccines that prevent severe disease for almost everyone.

The authors say that when P. flaciparum is cultured in vitro PfEMP1 loses its rosetting phenotype because it switches genes. The authors say that this can result in difficulties testing different strains of P. falciparum. You think you have an especially severe strain but it switches off the rosetting. Nevertheless, the authors say they have been able "to induce strain-transcending antibodies by immunization with a small number of PfEMP1 NTS-DBLα recombinant proteins". They got these antibodies in rabbits, but if they can make them we should be able to also. Humans are like rabbits, hopping around a lot, always worried about predators. In our case the predators are usually other humans.

I know I'm going back on my previous statements against animal testing and using data obtained from it, which is hypocritical of me. Hopefully these authors treated their rabbits like royalty at all times when they weren't jabbing them with needles. I would say they should be set free into the wild after helping with science, but the wild can be brutal for rabbits, especially if our cat is nearby.

The authors reason that the antibodies they got to NTS-DBLα "block rosetting by directly interfering with the receptor-ligand interaction between PfEMP1 and erythrocyte receptors." That's what I would have guessed. The NST-DBLα antigens that they got sound like great ingredients for a malaria vaccine. They haven't been tested on humans yet but hopefully soon

The next group of authors tested cross-reactivity of NTS-DBL1α to different strains of P. flaciparum malaria with different PfEMP1 adhesion molecules. They got antibodies to PfEMP1 by immunizing rats and goats with three different types of NTS-DBL1α, which they made in E. coli bacteria (34). They got the antibodies but found they did not get "extensive cross-reactivity in heterologus parasite strains." Bit of a disappointment there. But the authors aren't terribly discouraged. They suggest that "a combination of distinct DBL1α-domains in a possible multimeric vaccine against severe malaria could overcome the problem of low cross-reactivity." I said the same thing several lines back if you remember. To emphasize how different PfEMP1 types can be from one another how about this little fact from the authors: that its size can be anywhere from 200-400kDa. So some PfEMP1 types are about twice the size of others. Nevertheless, you figure there's probably some conserved stuff in there. If not, get a bunch of antigens for a vaccine or vaccines.

There seems to be some disappointing news from the authors of the next article, Ghumra and Khunrae et al. They were able to raise very effective antibodies that prevented rosetting to a high degree to a single type of rosetting malaria. Not only did they prevent rosetting well, they helped induce phagocytosis of infected erythrocytes. But those antibodies didn't work for 5 other types of rosetting malaria (35). So there was no cross-reactivity, at least as far as they tested. That's the bad news. The authors, who were no doubt hoping to find a single antigen that gave immunity to all rosetting, suggest combining the antigen they used with other antigens that will reduce rosetting in other varieties of malaria.

Unfortunately antigens tested by other researchers didn't seem to prevent rosettes as well as the one that Ghumra and Khunrae et al. found. Gumra and Khunrae et al. say that it could be that the other researchers results were better than they thought, since Ghumra and Khunae et al. used a rosette inhibition assay that was 10 times more sensitive than those used in earlier studies. They also suggest that their recombinant proteins fit better onto the NTS-DBL1α of the parasite. There seems to be a limited number of rosetting malarial types according to the authors, but maybe they're all able to make rosettes under the right conditions, like maybe hyperparasitemia.

The authors actually tried a number of different antibodies on the particular strain of malarial PfEMP1 they were working on and all of the antibodies inhibited rosettes to some extent. But none of them apparently worked for other malarial strains. On the other hand, the authors say that a different strain, Var 2CSA, has a PfEMP1 that is well conserved across other strains but there's been difficulty raising good rosette-disrupting antibodies to this PfEMP1. So maybe there still is hope for a rosette-inhibiting vaccine with relatively few malarial proteins. According to this article, it seems that past researchers have had trouble making good antibodies to the PfEMP1 varieties they were working on. Maybe as people learn more about how to get good antibodies we'll get some that cross-react more. Maybe these authors, who seem to be able to make excellent antibodies, should try working with the Var2CSA variety's PfEMP1. Maybe they'd hit the jackpot and could start shopping for Porches.

The authors of the next article, Cockburn et al., reason that the CR1 receptor (complement receptor 1) is the main rosetting receptor on non-parasitized red blood cells, and that CR1 deficiency gives resistance to cerebral malaria (36). They say that in Papua New Guinea around 80% of the people have CR1 deficiency. They add that in southeast Asia rosetting is not associated with severe malaria and that it could be because many people there have CR1 deficiency, which prevents rosetting to a large extent.

They also say that humans can have 50-1200 CR1s per red blood cell and that anything under 200 results in "greatly reduced rosetting". Apparently malaria isn't the massive killer in southeast Asia that it is in sub-Saharan Africa. Maybe P. falciparum malaria started infecting humans in New Guinea and southeast Asia, and by now the populations have evolved and acquired more resistance to the disease, including fewer CR1 receptors.

On the other hand, African population have acquired the sickle-cell trait, which protects them to some extent, but it doesn't affect anywhere near 80% of the population. I just looked it up. Sickle cell trait reaches 25-30% frequency in parts of Western Africa (37), which leaves lots of people unprotected. If you had up to 80% of healthy adults with the sickle cell trait you'd have lots of cases of sickle cell disease in the next generation.

Cockburn et al. say that one of the main features of α thalassemia is CR1 deficiency, that the malaria resistance that α thalassemia confers is not only due to small red blood cells, but also to low numbers of CR1 on the red blood cells. They note that α thalassemic red blood cells are only 15% smaller in surface area but have 50% fewer CR1 receptors.

CR1 receptors are probably the major rosetting receptor. The authors mention some CR1 polymorphisms in African populations, but they aren't nearly as prevalent as low-CR1 is in Papua New Guinea. Maybe P. falciparum started infecting humans there and then spread, giving that population more time to evolve ways to survive the disease.

The authors say that other red blood cell receptors only form weak rosettes but that CR1 forms strong ones that are more likely to clog microvessels. The authors say that fatality rates are still high for severe malaria even when intensive care is available. They suggest soluble recombinant CR1 as a therapy for severe malaria and they like the idea of an anti-rosetting vaccine. I would add, go for the CR1 to PfEMP1 rosettes, if it's possible to find that part of the PfEMP1. The vaccine is the way to go. Even with intensive care, if you show up to the hospital with severe malaria there's a good chance you'll die. Soluble CR1 would probably save lives, but if a lot of your blood cells are already rosetted and stuck in a micro blood vessel somewhere it might be too late for that. Best to head it off with vaccines.

Since there doesn't seem to be an anti-rosetting vaccine ready for humans yet, although it shouldn't take long, I thought maybe there's something a person could buy cheaply over the counter that would help keep blood moving in the tiny blood vessels. Soluble CR1 sounds great but I doubt if you can even get it at most hospitals and it almost surely needs to be taken intravenously. My brief search turned up ginseng. According to the authors of an article on the subject, ginseng induces the production of nitric oxide (NO) which "has known beneficial effects on the cardiovascular system (38)." They say that NO enhances "vasorelaxation". This could help keep blood vessels unclogged since they tend to be wider when relaxed.

The authors say that ginseng "inhibits the

expression of endothelial adhesion molecules." That's a good thing for malaria. The fewer infected red blood cells that cling to the cells lining blood vessels the better. As you recall, endothelial cells can be destroyed by infected red blood cells that are stuck to them, which can cause the blood vessel to clog. The authors say that not only does ginseng protect the endothelial cells that are there, it also promotes endothelial cell proliferation.

The authors did their experiments with Korean red ginseng water extract. This is probably not as readily available as ginseng, which here in the U.S. you can get at most grocery stores. I can see where a liquid form of ginseng might get into the bloodstream sooner. The only kind I've ever had was in capsules. Some energy drinks claim to have ginseng in them. Maybe some drinks with healthy amounts of liquid ginseng might be helpful for people with severe malaria, although I'm guessing that present energy drinks are not the answer. They usually contain caffeine, a vasoconstrictor. The authors also note that ginsenosides have been known to inhibit the release of inflammatory cytokines, which might also help keep blood vessels clear. They don't mention malaria at all, but from what the authors say about ginseng's effects, you might suspect it could help with some severe cases of the disease. Ginseng is made from a plant that grows in a variety of conditions and is already in production. The authors say that it has been used as an oriental folk medicine for thousands of years. Maybe if ginseng was found to be beneficial for severe malaria a ginseng drink or two might save lives in Africa.

Another way to increase NO in the blood is to inhale it. This would probably lead to increases in plasma NO faster than sending ginseng through the digestive system. You could possibly get a pressurized can of it or a tank, which are items that are not readily available over the counter right now. The authors of one article about inhaled NO tested it on mice that were fed high fat diets and then given transfusions of blood that had been stored for a long time. The authors say that stored blood, rather than fresh blood, causes vascular problems at least some of which are caused by lack of NO (39). They say that when blood is stored hemoglobin leaks out of the red blood cells and reacts with the NO, converting it to something else, which makes NO less available than it should be. The authors say that the effects of free hemoglobin in the blood are vasoconstriction, inflammation and platelet activation, all of which tend to reduce blood flow. During malaria you have red blood cells being broken down by the immune system which frees hemoglobin to react with available NO, removing NO from the blood. It sounds like NO deficiency is probably partly responsible for the clogging of blood vessels with severe malaria.

The authors mention platelet activation as an effect of free hemoglobin in the blood. You want platelets to be activated against parasites if you've got malaria, but you don't want them over-activated to where they stop blood flow in small vessels of your brain. The authors found that inhaled NO helped reduce vasoconstriction and inflammation in their experimental mice. If it could do that for humans with severe malaria maybe it could save lives.

Hopefully, after the experiments the mice were freed into a beautiful sunny field where cats are not allowed in. The researchers ought to drop off some high quality mouse food for them occasionally too.

The authors of the next article say that NO is "a well-known pro-angiogenic molecule" which can cause the formation of new blood vessels as well as repair the old ones (40). The authors say that nitrite, which is an oxidation product of NO, does about the same things as NO and might be good to give to people with myocardial, liver, kidney and brain ischemia / re-perfusion injuries. In other words, if lack of blood flow to these areas is causing problems, nitrite has been shown to help.

Dietary NO is good too. You can get this by eating leafy green vegetables such as spinach or lettuce and beet roots also have a lot of it. Maybe people who have eaten plenty of leafy green vegetables in the not too distant past are less likely to get severe malaria because they have more NO in them. Maybe leafy green vegetables would be good to eat even after you get malaria.

The authors caution that even if you eat the right veggies, if you don't have them in your mouth for a while to interact with the bacteria in your mouth, you won't get the NO. You'll get inorganic nitrate which apparently isn't anywhere near as good. The authors say that if you wash your mouth out with a bactericidal mouthwash every day you kill the good bacteria that convert inorganic nitrate to NO. This will result in an NO deficiency and your blood vessels and organs can suffer as a result. So don't use too much mouthwash, at least the bactericidal kind. My father used a lot of Listerine mouthwash, the old fashioned kind, which they still sell a lot of, tan colored. He had chronic heart problems for the last ten years of his life and died of a heart attack at age 71. One wonders if the Listerine might have hurt him. Maybe those people you meet who have really smelly breath have excellently perfused vital organs.

Other things that the authors say that NO or nitrite can do include lower blood pressure, inhibit platelet aggregation, increase exercise tolerance, and improve mitrochondrial efficiency. Those all sound good for malaria sufferers except inhibit platelet aggregation. In some cases inhibiting platelets might be good for a malaria sufferer if platelets are clogging up vessels. But if they are helping get rid of parasites and parasitized red blood cells, you don't want to inhibit that too much, if possible. So this whole idea of more NO or nitrite for malaria may be a good thing, but in some cases maybe not. Either way, keep working on vaccines. You get two or three of the right vaccines and you're probably immune from severe malaria. We've just got to find out what those vaccines are.

The authors of the next article say that experimental cerebral malaria in mice is partially prevented by the NO donor DPTA-NO in high doses (41). They say the only big problem with it is that it causes a major drop in blood pressure. They tried to avoid this by lowering the dose of DPTA-NO and combining it with sildenafil, which is Viagra. The authors say that sildenafil prolongs the effects of NO in your body rather than causing more to be made, which they figure might lessen the drop in blood pressure.

The authors are serious about cerebral malaria not only because it kills 18-30% of people who get it, but also because they figure it causes cognitive disabilities in about 30% of the children who get it. That would suggest that there are lots of people in Africa with brain problems, which would add to that continent's long list of problems, which also includes exploitation by more powerful countries to the north whose "foreign aide" consists mostly of military hardware and rapacious loans. Just what they need. The authors add that there is very little long-term support or treatment for neurological problems caused by malaria. In short, malaria is a big problem for Africa.

The authors give a nice progression of events for cerebral malaria: it starts with vascular constriction, then goes to vascular occlusion, endothelial activation with intravascular inflammation, microhemorrhages and eventual vascular collapse. In your brain this translates into more and more neurons dying. The whole mess is at least partly caused by low NO bioavailability. They also mention the fact that NO is destroyed during malaria by free-floating hemoglobin which is in the blood because of hemolysis of parasitized red blood cells. This description makes it sound like any strain of P. falciparum malaria that can load up your blood with parasites is capable of causing cerebral malaria, as opposed to the idea that only some strains cause it. The number of parasites in your blood probably depends on the state of your immune system. If your immune system has no previous experience of malaria or any of its antigens it's more likely cerebral malaria will develop. This suggest that vaccines might prevent cerebral malaria by giving the immune system some readiness for the disease. In fact even a vaccine without malarial antigens might be enough to put the immune system on alert thus putting up a better fight against malaria when it does come.

The authors say that one large injection of DPTA-NO prevents cerebral malaria in mice, even though it only lasts for 4 hours or less in the bloodstream. They're talking about mice here, but it might work for humans too, which would be great. The sildenefil DPTA-NO combination sounds good too, but you probably have to get to a hospital or clinic to get it. If it takes a long time to get to the hospital or if they make you fill out endless sheets of questions and promises to pay, you might still get cerebral malaria.

The authors also mention that the nitric oxide synthase enzyme might be in short supply due to cerebral malaria. The parasites might have a way of getting rid of this molecule which is important for making NO. Maybe so, but it seems more likely that NO gets eaten up by free hemoglobin. The authors say that sildenafil alone doesn't prevent cerebral malaria probably because there is so little NO for the drug to enhance the activity of. They say that sildenafil doesn't work for erectile dysfunction when there's not much NO to start with. The authors have some interesting insights and give reason for hope for effective medicine against cerebral malaria in the near future, but no reason to stop working on vaccines and to make some of them available immediately.

The authors of the next article say that less than 1% of P. falciparum malaria cases become life threatening. They say the innate immune response, which is non-specific, usually fights the infection long enough for a specific immune response to develop. This article is about platelets and their importance in malaria fighting. They are non-specific yet crucial parasite killers say the authors, who add that they have direct parasite killing functions and their number and mass are far greater than all leukocytes combined. I've always thought of them as little circulating pieces of solidified goop ready to turn slimy and gum up anything that isn't supposed to be in the circulatory system, but the authors tell us that platelets can also produce oxygen-free radicals and microbicidal peptides. The authors maintain that if platelets can do their non-specific

65

policing job against malaria, malaria is almost always defeated.

They say that malaria is accompanied by thrombocytopenia, in other words, lack of platelets, which mirrors increasing parasite mass. Maybe the platelets get used up after a while trying to fight the gazillions of blood-born parasites. Or maybe the immune system cuts back on platelet production to keep from clogging blood vessels. Nevertheless, the authors say that platelets protect against malarial blood infection and that mice with platelet deficiencies are more susceptible to infection and have higher numbers of viable parasites. The authors say that mice given aspirin, a well-known platelet inhibitor, have reduced survival of malaria. They add that thrombocytopenia is associated with poor outcome for P. falciparum malaria. You want those platelets to be there working, usually, right up to the time they help clog up the blood vessels in your brain.

The authors remind us that platelets are often found at sites of infected erythrocyte sequestration in cerebral malaria. The authors also mention a review that found that they couldn't tell if aspirin is good or bad for malaria. It sounds to me like it might be a matter of timing. Early on in the disease, forget it. While the blood is still flowing well let the platelets do their microbe-killing job. But if signs of cerebral malaria become evident, maybe some aspirin would help keep the blood flowing in the brain and other vital organs.

The authors say that sub-Saharan African populations might be more susceptible to severe infection by Plasmodium falciparum because of a missing receptor on red blood cells (42). This receptor, called Duffy, enabled P. vivax to enter red blood cells. P. vivax might have been more deadly than it is now and the genetic loss of the Duffy receptor would have defeated P. vivax. The authors say that in central and western Africa almost everyone is Duffy-negative.

Unfortunately the Duffy receptor is needed for signaling that enables platelets to bind and kill parasites, say the authors. They figure that P. falciparum is a more recent disease in Africa and that it is not as deadly in other parts of the world where it is common, such as southern Asia and South America. Even so, it seems to me that populations as exposed to P. falciparum malaria as those in central and western Africa would not have retained a mutation that put them at a disadvantage against the disease for very long, especially when the Duffy gene is available in other nearby populations.

My guess is that if they are close to 100% Duffy negative in those areas there might actually be an advantage to being Duffy negative with respect to malaria. P. falciparum malaria has certainly had enough time to change the genetics of sub-Saharan populations. The sickle cell trait is evidence of that. If Duffy negative was making people in that part of the world more susceptible to death by malaria I would guess that by now in those areas most people would be Duffy positive. As you recall, some authors that we reviewed earlier found that NO and its effects could enhance resistance to malaria. NO suppresses the effects of platelets to some extent. Maybe people with very high parasite loads who appear to be asymptomatic are often those who are Duffy negative. Maybe platelets are responsible to a large extent for clogging up blood vessels in the brain. What could happen with Duffy-negative people is that their immune systems don't do well at fighting the parasites to begin with, parasite load becomes very high, but since there is little platelet-caused coagulation, their organs stand a good chance of surviving the disease until the specific immune system finally adapts to the parasites. The next time they get the disease they have some extra immunity and a better chance at survival.

The authors say that malaria is more deadly in Africa than anywhere else, suggesting that Duffy-negative is the reason. But there could be many reasons for that, such as poor health care systems, poor quality education, and lower per-capita income, to name a few. Nevertheless, their article is very interesting. Whether or not Duffy-positive or Duffy-negative gives an advantage against malaria, we're not going to change the genetics of human populations very soon. Better to get the vaccines out there in the hope of fending off deadly malaria. A person might still get malaria, but be less likely to die or be neurologically messed up from it with a good vaccine or two or three.

Artemisinin and Other Drugs

This next section is about Artemisinin, and other drugs for malaria, as you may have guessed. Artemisinin is very effective but it might not be in ten years if malaria parasites become resistant to it. The author of the first article in this section we'll look at considers today's anti-malarial drugs a bridge to a good vaccine or a single dose drug cure (43). Well, the kind of vaccine he hopes for, one that will prevent the disease in almost all cases might never get here. Nevertheless, vaccines might keep severe disease from developing. In many cases anti-malarial drugs can do that too.

The author says that not only does malaria cause about a million deaths a year, 90% of them children, but 25% of adults in endemic countries are unable to work because of malaria. That's a huge impact on these countries, not to mention the people who live there. That would suggest that everyone there spends about a quarter of the year feeling bad because of the disease. That's a lot of sick days. If the vaccines we have are not able to completely prevent malaria, which is likely to be the case for quite a while, drugs may be able to cut down on the sick days as well as deaths and neurological complications.

The author says that quinine was used against malaria from the 17th century to the 1940s, when other drugs were developed that had fewer side effects. The stuff can kill you, but one of the other possible side effects that might be disturbing is loss of hearing and deafness.

Wikipedia says it's reversible once you get off the stuff, but who knows? Maybe that's just what the doctors tell you to keep you from going nuts and tearing up their clinic. A woman I know has been on hydroxychloroquine for a while for arthritis pain. I always have to repeat whatever I say to her, often more than once.

Many people still use quinine because it's cheap says the author. He says that in the late 1940s chloroquine was introduced and then a bunch of other drugs, mostly quinolones but some others too. He mentions half a dozen others including mefloquine, which unfortunately can cause "serious neuropsychiatric problems". Maybe that's how the stuff works, by driving parasites nuts. The author adds that many of these drugs have limited effectiveness due to parasite resistance. They're all going to become less effective the more they're used. That might happen with vaccines too, but with vaccines you've got lots of parasite antigens to target with new vaccines.

Artemisinin comes from the sweet wormwood plant Artemisia annua the author tells us. The old alcoholic drink absinthe was made with wormwood. Maybe it helped some people with malaria back when it was still legal. The Chinese discovered artemisinin in 1972. The author says it causes a major kill-off of malarial parasites in a short time, since it has a half-life of 2-5 hours, patients feel lots better, think they're cured, don't take any more of the 14 day supply of artemisinin and in a short time the disease is back because all it takes is a few survivors to give rise to massive numbers of parasites, as we know. Artemisinin based combination therapy (ACT) is the preferred prescription now, which only requires that you stay with it for 3 days, says the author. It's got some quinolones in it to attack the little beasts from that angle too.

The author says that even a mere three days is too long to ensure that sufferers take their meds in some areas. Maybe lack of money is a problem. Or maybe people don't believe the doctors, nurses or pharmacists. I've certainly run into doctors I didn't trust. The author says that ACTs are expensive and rural folks shy away from them for that reason and that counterfeit drugs are a problem. He adds that a vaccine would be the ideal solution. I would modify that to say the ideal vaccine would be the ideal solution, but any malaria vaccine adopted in the near future is unlikely to be ideal or perfect. There will be many people who still get the disease but probably fewer who die or suffer life-altering brain damage from it.

The ideal anti-malarial drug would be a single dose cure, says the author. I would add that it should be super-cheap or free. But even then, some people would consider the walk or ride to the clinic too much trouble and wind up with severe or deadly disease. Of course there will be abstainers from vaccines too.

The author says that researchers have synthesized endoperoxides, which is what artemisinin is, that have "greater efficacy" than artemisinin itself, but the big obstacles are time and money for clinical trials. Clinical trials are important but hopefully it's not another of these 50 year obstacle courses. Money shouldn't be an issue. Tell the U.S. federal government to divert funds from the making of one or two of its high-tech jet fighters which we don't use anymore anyway because of Washington's love of drones. The cash problem would be solved. The author says that these new antimalarials should be excellent and that "rock-bottom pricing" is required. I agree. If the U.S. could forgo one of its many wars of choice this would be easily attainable. The author says that techniques for growing Artemesia plants are improving. They only take 6 months to mature but it's still a tricky crop says the author. He adds that he recently published a cheap way to synthesize artemisinin with "widely available commodity chemicals." This article gives plenty of reason for hope, but there are already signs of resistance to artemisinin.

If artemisinin's anti-malarial effect fades hopefully some new synthetic endoperoxides similar to it will still do the job. A more recent article states that fully synthetic endoperoxides are now in pre-clinical and clinical trials (44). They say researchers are hoping that OZ439 will be a single dose cure. It sounds like they've really got artemisinin figured out but the authors tell us the mechanism of action is still debated.

The authors of the next article write about the problems of counterfeit antimalarial drugs in Africa. They say it was bad in the pre-artemisinin combination therapy days and is still going on (45). That's what happens when the drugs people need cost a significant amount of money. Antimalarials should be cheap or free or there will be counterfeiters. The authors say that counterfeit drugs probably helped lead to parasite resistance against previous antimalarials, such as sulphadoxine-pyramethamine and chloroquine. This can happen because counterfeit drugs often contain sub-theraputic amounts of the drugs they purport to be. Sometimes non-counterfeit drugs degrade due to heat or sitting around too long to where there is sub-standard levels of active ingredients, which can also lead to resistance against the drug, say the authors.

They say there has been "an alarming increase in reports of poor quality ACTs" as well as other antimalarial drugs in Africa. This could easily lead to people needlessly dying of malaria or suffering a severe case of it. The authors give an example of a counterfeit drug that contained sildenafil, which is Viagra. It might help with some cases of malaria due to its NO-enhancing effects, and having a boner might distract you from your suffering for a while, but it's not supposed to be there.

The authors say that pollen analyses of some counterfeit drugs found that they came from east Asia. Apparently pollen makes a good adulterant in capsules. It's powdery and all you have to do is sweep some up off your patio if it's that time of year. The authors say that some production and packaging takes place in Africa. That's understandable considering that the World Health Organization figures that 30% of countries in Africa have no or hardly any drug regulation, and only 3 African countries have WHO-approved drug testing labs, say the authors. They add that the situation is so bad that it might be endangering clinical trials.

To end their article on a happy note, the authors say that drug-testing technology has improved a lot lately and portable testing units should help eliminate the bad drugs. My issue would be, if a person buys a substandard antimalarial drug because it's cheaper when they wouldn't have bought the more high quality drug that has the claimed amount of active ingredients, and that person still receives some benefit from the substandard drug, is that really so bad, especially if the substandard drug saved her life? Sure, it probably didn't cure her but she's still alive. The only way out of a quandary like this is to have super-cheap or free antimalarials or vaccines that vastly reduce the probability of severe or deadly malaria.

The authors of the next article were interested in artemisinin drug quality in Ghana and what they found was that it is pretty good. They tested 33 drugs from 16 shops and only found one drug sample that had less than 80% of its purported active ingredients. That's not too bad. They say that artemisinin monotherapy were about 21% of the drugs they collected; the rest were ACT. The authors were surprised drug quality was so high. They say ACT combines artemisinin with some other more slow-acting drug.

They add that artemisinin resistance has been reported in Cambodia. Hopefully it hasn't reached anywhere else yet. This article was written in 2010. The authors say that artemisinin cost 10 times more than other antimalarials and ACT is even more expensive. They called prices "extremely high" and "well above the cost that most ordinary Ghanaians can afford", although there was supposed to be some kind of drug subsidy on the way. The authors say that resistance to chloroquine happened in parts of east Africa in the 1980s and to Sulphadoxine-pyramethamine in the 1990s.

An idea that I had that is probably impractical is to quit using an old antimalarial, like chloroquine, completely for 10 years. By that time resistance to it among parasites might be lost. Chloroquine resistance might require an extra expenditure of energy or the toting around of extra proteins. If these became unnecessary they might be lost. Then after 10 years you might find that chloroquine is once again a very effective antimalarial. The problems are that you have many countries and surely some parasites that are not yet resistant to it. It's still probably saving some lives. And also, it might take longer than 10 years.

The authors found that drug quality was good from both licensed and unlicensed sellers. That's encouraging. One hopes that the new drug subsidies in that country will enable the average citizen to buy the best antimalarials. Something tells me they are probably still expensive now and will be for as long as they are still effective. Encouraging as this study is, it's certainly no reason not to make vaccines available as soon as possible. Most Ghanaians probably still cannot afford effective antimalarial drugs.

The authors of the next article say that up to 50% of artemisinin-based drugs have been found to be counterfeit in southeast Asia, especially Cambodia (46). They say that many have died of curable malaria because they got phony drugs. The authors have found two color reactions that can indicate the presence of artemisinin and the concentration of it by the depth of the colors in the reaction. They say the tests are cheap, accurate and easy to use. Maybe the authors should say the tests should be cheap. If a corporation decides to market these things they're going to want to make as much profit as possible. Maybe the authors should take a business course or two and market their testing kits themselves rather than allowing the capitalist system to handle the job. The authors add that counterfeit artemisinin has been found in 6 sub-Saharan countries. The number is probably that low because they couldn't afford to do tests in the other 40 or so. The authors note a lack of dedicated lab facilities in sub-Saharan Africa.

They say that a semi-synthetic artemisinin drug also tested positive with their test kit. That's good, since the synthesis of artemisinin-like drugs is probably the main direction that malaria drug invention is headed. The authors mention that even if you start with a good quality artemisinin drug it can easily be degraded by light, heat, and humidity, another good reason for rigorous testing of drugs, and also another reason to keep working on vaccines and get them on the market now. As you can see, there are many ways that you can die from a curable case of malaria. Wait a little too long for the degraded or counterfeit drug you payed good money for to make you feel better and your wife may soon go pine box shopping.

The authors of the next article mention a documented case of a 23 year-old man in Burma who died because he relied on fake artesunate, an artemisinin-derived drug (47). The authors tested 24 drug samples from Kenya and the Democratic Republic of the Congo (DR Congo). All samples had some of the purported active ingredients in them but 7 had under 95% of the active ingredient. 90% doesn't sound too bad but 10% would be. The authors say malaria is the number one killer disease in the third world, especially sub-Saharan Africa. They say it kills 18% of children under 5 years old each year. I would guess that if it did kill 18% of young children that the death toll would be over a million. Who know? Maybe it is.

The authors say you can often find cheap ineffective drug copies next to good name brand drugs in the same pharmacy, from the same wholesalers. They say the cheap copies are for people who can't afford the good stuff. Once again I think we are confronted with what is apparently the scientific community's definition of "ineffective" treatment for malaria. They consider the treatment ineffective if it does not cure the patient. I would suggest that if the treatment kept the patient from dying or suffering severely that the treatment was effective.

The authors themselves say that all the samples they took had some artemesinin-derived drugs in them. Maybe some samples didn't have enough to cure the patient for the little money spent, and fell below the 95% active ingredient threshold the authors were worried about, but saved lives and brain cells of people who couldn't afford the expensive stuff that was over the 95% threshold. If a drug saves your life even though it's cheap and not exactly what its label says it is and doesn't cure you, I say it's still an effective drug. Until the money-grubbers back off and the high-powered drugs that the scientists love become affordable for everyone, I don't think it's bad that the less powerful drugs are available for people who can't afford anything else. It's undoubtedly saved lives.

The authors say that in the big cities in most parts of Africa artemisinin-derivatives can easily be gotten without a prescription. The authors say most of the "sub-therapeutic" drugs they found came from either India or China, because in those countries they regulate drugs for domestic use but not for export. Once again, is a dose of artemisinin "sub-therapeutic" if it kills enough parasites to save your life, even if it doesn't completely cure you? No, it's still therapeutic.

The authors say that in Kenya all the analyzed drugs had an official sales license even though half were "sub-standard". I think "sub-standard" is a more accurate term for these drugs than "sub-therapeutic". They say 71% of the dry powders they tested were substandard, which is too bad because these powders are specifically made for children. That's the age group that really gets hit by malaria. I just read yesterday that the U.S. has decided to upgrade their nuclear weapons arsenal to the tune of a trillion dollars. A small fraction of that wasted money could supply the malaria endemic areas of the world with cheap high quality artemisinin-derived drugs.

The author of this next article says that not only might your antimalarial drugs contain little if any artemisinin, they might contain toxic ingredients, such as metamizole, which can lead to bone marrow failure, melamine, which can cause lethal urinary lithiasis, or safrole, which can cause liver cancer and was used as a flavoring agent back in the 1950s (48). Death by kidney stones sounds horrible. That would make a good movie. A guy almost dies of kidney stones after taking counterfeit antimalarials, then after he recovers he hunts down the counterfeiters. At the end we're treated to a prolonged torture to death scene for the bad guys. If you knew someone who died of kidney stones after taking antimalarial medicine you might elect to take your chances on the disease, even if you had the money and the drugs were available.

You might expect the packaging to look like an amateurish copy, but the author says that's not so. The counterfeit drugs can be very well packaged with "identical holograms, batch numbers, expiry dates, blisters and tablets looking absolutely genuine". Drugs for malaria? No thanks, I think this is just a mild case.

The author says a recent case in east Africa lead to the arrests of fake drug manufacturers, wholesalers, and retail pharmacists, as well as the confiscation of several billion dollars worth of fake antimalarials. The authors point out that counterfeit drugs could lead researchers to wrongly conclude that resistance to the good drugs is spreading. People whose lives could be saved or whose children's lives could be saved by good antimalarials might think, "Why bother? Those drugs don't work anyway." The author says the problem of counterfeit antimalarials won't be solved until genuine antimalarials are given to the populations of sub-Saharan Africa for free. I would say, make that anywhere else the disease is endemic also. The authors quote an article in PLOS Medicine that found that 30 to 35% of antimalarials in southeast Asia were counterfeit. Make the drugs free. Have the U.S. pay for them out of their Regime-Change with Mass Murder budget. Also, start rolling out the malaria vaccines. With a good vaccine or two the demand for antimalarial drugs might go down, causing them to become cheaper and making drug counterfeiting less worth the effort.

The authors of a recent review say that the high price of genuine antimalarials is the reason for the counterfeit market (49). They suggest governments lower taxes on the drugs and "encourage domestic manufacture of good quality and affordable generic drugs." Those are good ideas but they don't sound like enough to discourage fake drug production in the near future. On the other hand, there are vaccines now that are known to reduce the risk of getting malaria.

Breastfeeding and Malaria

This next section is about how breast feeding can make your child more resistant to malaria. Apparently the breast milk of women who have had malaria themselves, which includes just about everyone in sub-Saharan Africa, has some protection against malaria as well as other diseases. Mothers everywhere, if they're more or less healthy, should breastfeed their babies. It seems to give the youngster a better shot at staying healthy and having a good life. The benefits might actually last a lifetime if the child winds up getting allergies or asthma that she wouldn't have had if her mother had fed her mother's milk. Of course if the non-breastfed child contracts a case of malaria that kills her that wouldn't have been deadly had she been breastfed, that would make a big difference in her life.

The authors of the first article in this section say that children who had early complimentary feeding, which is food not from mommy's breasts, had lower weight for age at 3 months, 6 months, and 9 months of age (50). These kids also had more respiratory infections and "marginally increased risk for eye infection and episodes of malaria." They call it marginally increased risk but later in the same article they say it was a significantly increased risk for both eye infection and malaria. They also say maternal illiteracy was associated with earlier feeding of complimentary foods. So maybe the mothers who give their children less breast milk aren't quite as smart or well informed as those that let the kids suck longer, which might mean other things the non-breastfeeding mothers do also cause their kids to be less healthy.

The authors say later complimentary feeding was associated with reduced infant morbidity and improved growth. They say the WHO figures kids should be breastfed for 6 months, at least. That's not just Africa, that's everywhere. A friend of mine has Crohn's disease, which is another one that's associated with non-breastfeeding. He seems to have some allergies too. I'm guessing he was never breastfed. He gets regular blood tests and doctor's check-ups for his Crohn's.

A woman I know well was never breastfed. She has asthma, another disease associated with not being breast fed. She's in her 50s and wakes up some nights with difficulty breathing and has to use an inhaler, which has a stimulant effect and keeps her up the rest of the night. She doesn't smoke. Going outside in the summer for her can be a problem because of her allergies. When she was a child few people if any knew the long-term benefits of breastfeeding. If you or your wife can't breastfeed your kid, consider finding a wet nurse or some source for mother's milk. It might really help your child a lot.

The authors say that in developing countries infants who aren't breastfed from birth to 5 months are 5 and 7 times more likely to die of diarrhea and pneumonia respectively. They add that breastfeeding could reduce deaths of children under 5 years old by 13%. That is a lot of children. But that doesn't take into account the children who survive but have serious long-term health problems that wouldn't have happened had they had the mother's milk. The authors say gastrointestinal infection is also more likely without mother's milk.

They say that adolescent pregnancies and poverty tend to push mothers away from breastfeeding. They say some mothers live in extreme poverty and that without "income generation initiatives" preaching to people about breastfeeding might not do much good. If a mother barely has enough to keep herself alive breastfeeding might not be possible.

The authors note that in parts of rural Malawi

25.6% of mothers are HIV positive. That is extremely sad. There's a 7% chance every year that the breastfeeding infant of an HIV positive mother will become HIV positive say the authors. In this case, it might be best not to breastfeed. But if you do and the kid doesn't get HIV, the little one definitely got some extra protection that might last a lifetime. If you only breastfeed the kid for 6 months that would cut the risk of transmitting the virus down to 3.5%, if I understand the authors correctly. Maybe that's why WHO only recommends 6 months of breastfeeding. Longer than that and the risk of HIV transmission becomes too high. I doubt if rural Malawians are much more HIV positive than other parts of sub-Saharan Africa. That area is loaded with the deadly virus. Basically what mother's milk does is transfer immunity to the young child. The goal of malaria vaccines it to enhance whatever immunity is already there. Better to have a strong immune response to begin with, but even if you don't, vaccines can help build up your immune system.

The next article says that several things lower the risk of severe malaria in a child, almost all relating to the mother: maternal education, mother's adequate knowledge about malaria, mother's use of mosquito bed nets, and breast feeding for at least 2 years (51). That's a lot of breast feeding, but it sounds like a great idea as long as the mother doesn't have HIV and can produce the milk. My guess is that any amount of breast feeding will give the child some protection against malaria, at least for a while.

The authors also seem to say that yellow fever vaccination protects against severe malaria. This looks like an example of a vaccine that stimulates the innate immune system. The part of the vaccine that induces a response specific to the yellow fever virus probably doesn't do any good against malaria. Even so, a strong innate immune response can apparently lessen the chances for severe malaria. It looks like you don't have to have any malarial antigens in a vaccine in order for it to offer some valuable protection. If you throw some malarial antigens in too, better still. Maybe it won't absolutely prevent malaria, which the "scientific community" has been holding out for for decades now, but it will save lives.

The next article finds antibodies in Nigerian mother's milk to the various stages of P. falciparum (52). They also found in-vitro growth inhibition against P. falciparum by breastmilk constituents lactoferrin and secretory IgA. If lactoferrin suppresses growth of malaria parasites maybe it should be included in infant formulas. Apparently it's not the easiest stuff to produce. Wikipedia says it can either be purified from milk or produced recombinantly. The latter would be best, but it's not like you just whip together a few chemicals in a beaker. Wikipedia says lactoferrin is part of the innate immune system and has bactericidal, fungicidal, anti-viral and anticarcinogenic effects. They say that colostrum (first milk) has the highest concentration, followed by human, then cow milk. Sounds like human milk is good for a young child to have.

Being a vegan myself, I might take a look at the health food store and see if they have any that's produced recombinantly. If they get it from cow's milk forget it. I don't want to support the dairy-torture of unwanted veal calves to death system. You shouldn't either. Boycott diary completely.

An article about lactoferrin says that bovine milk contains only a tiny fraction of the lactoferrin that human milk does, especially colostrum, which has about 7mg/mL and bovine milk has 0.02-0.2mg/mL (53). That's a big difference. The authors say that only bovine produced lactoferrin was available when they wrote their article in 1997. Hopefully large amounts are now being produced recombinantly. The authors say that until then (1997) most infant formulas did not contain lactoferrin. Considering the large amounts of lactoferrin in human milk, I think it's safe to say that infant formulas should have large amounts of it too. It would save lives of some children who would otherwise die of malaria and who knows how many other diseases.

G. Chirico et al., authors of the next article, say

that breastfeeding has activity against "several viruses, bacteria, and protozoa" (54). They add that the human immune system "is completed only several years after birth." So breastfeeding gives the child some protection during a time when the child's immune system is still under construction. The authors say that neonates have "increased susceptibility to various infections", especially pre-terms, who have higher incidence of infection, sepsis, morbidity, mortality, and neurological problems. They say breastfeeding maintains the maternal-fetal immunological link.

They say kids breastfed over 4 months have protection against severe respiratory tract infections, ear infections, and urinary tract infections. Maybe kids who are not breastfed who drink formula with cows mild have some protection against hoof and mouth disease that they don't really need. The authors say that if you're in the market to buy some mother's milk get the unpasteurized kind. Pasteurization might kill or destroy some of the good stuff.

G. Chirico et al. say that in developed countries if the mother is HIV positive they advise against breastfeeding. I've read that the HIV virus is pretty fragile. I wonder if Pasteurization might destroy it. I just looked it up. "Flash-heating" of mother's milk apparently "successfully inactivated the free-floating virus"(55). It looks like a double boiler set up with milk in a jar in the middle of a pot of boiling water. Apparently you don't boil the milk or anything close to it. Just heat it up. The author says the technique could be used at mother's milk banks. Hopefully the milk would retain a lot of its immune bolstering effects after the heat up.

G. Chirico et al. say that in places where not breast feeding is difficult HIV infected mothers should breast feed for the first 6 months. After that you should try to figure out something else to give the youngster or risk giving her HIV. G. Chirico and friends say that neonates lack immunoglobulin A (IgA) but that there's lots of it in colostrum and still pretty much in regular mother's milk.

They add that IgA$_2$ is more resistant to digestive acid and bacterial proteases. So you figure a bunch of this will get into the child's bloodstream. Good deal!

They mention that lactoferrin, which you'll recall is present in large amounts in colostrum and regular mother's milk, also resists breakdown in the digestive system. The authors say that lactoferrin also has epithelial growth promoting activities. That might help junior recover faster from cuts and scrapes and have healthier skin all around, which is part of the innate immune system. Maybe a tumbler of mother's milk would do a lot of us some good. Maybe lactoferrin would be good for someone with road rash from a motorcycle accident.

The authors say that 4 month-old children who weren't breastfed were found to have smaller thymuses, which might reflect a weaker immune system. The authors say that breastfed kids have "a better developed response" to vaccines, such as those for influenza, oral poliovirus, tetanus, and diphtheria. They add that breastfeeding offers long-term protection against allergy development, insulin-dependent diabetes, Crohn's disease, ulcerative colitis, and tumors in infancy. Ladies, please do your children a huge favor and breastfeed them. The government should do more to encourage breastfeeding. Not only should it be legal to breastfeed anywhere anytime, but fellow citizens should be encouraged to give the breastfeeding mom dollar bills. That's right. Stop what you're doing, pull out your wallet, get a dollar bill, and give it to the breastfeeding mom. It should become a firmly established custom in all parts of the world.

The authors say that most of the cytokines that are deficient in infants are found in healthy quantities in mother's milk. They go on to list a dozen or so. Not only are these cytokines present in mother's milk say the authors, but so are various immune cells that produce them. Maybe some day they'll figure out a way to make mother's milk without the mothers, in the factory. But it seems unlikely to happen in the near future. Maybe women can be stimulated hormonally to produce mother's milk in large quantities without having to have a baby, so we could have a lot more available to sell to mothers who can't breastfeed. But juicing up women with enough hormones to fool their breasts into thinking they've given birth when they weren't even pregnant might also cause problems.

Another group of authors found that boys who live in the city are less likely to suffer from asthma if they were breastfed more than 6 months (56). When I look at the chart with their numbers it looks like a pretty solid correlation between breastfeeding and avoiding asthma for girls too, but apparently the authors statistics program didn't give them a "significant" relationship. Even so, it looks like a strong tendency to me.

The authors say that a study from New Zealand found the children who were breastfed more than 4 weeks were more likely to get asthma. That's unexpected. I should probably look more closely at that one. Was it funded by the makers of infant formula? Even so, it seems likely that breastfeeding does protect children from malaria, especially if the mother has had the disease herself. Who knows? A specific antibody or two might make it into the bloodstream. Protection from breastmilk might help a child to survive malaria during the part of life when she is most vulnerable. Even so, if the youngster quits breastfeeding at 6 months of age there are unprotected years ahead, unless the child's immune system is given a head start on the disease through one or more malaria vaccines.

Nutrition and Malaria

This section is about nutrition, especially malnutrition, which is more common in sub-Saharan Africa and other malaria endemic areas than in many other parts of the world. The author of the first article says "promotion of exclusive breastfeeding is ranked as the most effective intervention for reducing the mortality of <5 year-olds.(57)" She goes on to say that less than 30% of children under 6 months old are exclusively breast fed. That's a low number, but it would be interesting to know how many are at least getting some mother's milk. For them I'd guess that some is better than none. The author says that a "lactation education" program in Ghana raised breastfeeding rates 100%. Sounds like a good thing, however recently an Ebola education team was slaughtered somewhere in west Africa. It's risky being an educator, someone who gets up in front of people and tells them things. Every now and then here in the U.S. you read about a professor who gets shot.

The author considered breastfeeding for its nutritional quality rather than its immune system enhancement. She says that pregnant and lactating women, infants and young children are most at risk for nutritional deficiencies. She points out "pervasive poverty" is found in sub-Saharan Africa. This is probably a major reason things are so screwed up in that part of the world. If people in sub-Saharan Africa had lots of cash they might have malaria vaccines to choose from by now. But the question is if they even get around to making a malaria vaccine available, who's going to pay for it? Drug companies want money. They have shareholders who demand cash. In places with pervasive poverty the people that need the vaccines probably won't be able to afford them. So who pays? The government? The U.N.? Rich philanthropists? None of the above?

Here's a piece of information from the author that tells you how bad health care in sub-Saharan Africa is: in that part of the world the chances of a woman dying of pregnancy-related causes is 1 in 16. In "industrialized countries" it's 1 in 4000. What a huge difference! The author says that in sub-Saharan Africa pregnancy is a life-threatening situation. Apparently so. To me this seems like another reason that vaccines are needed, because if you wait until people get malaria to treat them there's a good chance they won't get the treatment they need. Even if rapid treatment and high-quality care are essential it seems likely in that part of the world you won't get it.

It seems more possible to reduce the chances of severe disease with vaccines, which are given when the person is healthy with less effort on the part of the almost non-existent health care systems. The author figures that micro nutrients ground up and put in children's food could save lives. She says that the usual foods that non-nursing children usually get in that part of the world are "watery cereal porridges of low energy and nutrient densities." Yes, some crushed vitamins in there would probably help, and might help them fight off malaria more effectively too, although some nutrients might actually benefit the malaria parasites if you have the disease. More about that later. Hint: vitamin E might fall into that category. The author also recommends nutrition education for people in sub-Saharan Africa, and a push for dietary diversification. Sounds great if you can do it for not too much money and safely.

The authors of the next article say that malnutrition contributes to about 1/3 of child deaths worldwide but it's rarely listed as a direct cause (58). They say it can help ease kids into graves who have respiratory tract infections, including TB, diarrheal diseases, malaria, and anemia. In these underdeveloped countries where people have little education and health care in many places consists of the local herbal healer, the main weapon a person has to fight disease with is their own immune system. If that doesn't work properly because necessary nutrients are lacking you're in trouble.

The authors say that children under 5 years old are most at risk for malnutrition. What a coincidence! Those are the same age people who malaria usually kills. Maybe these guys are on to something. They rightly wonder why people in that part of the world aren't getting the food they need. They say that distribution obstacles should be dealt with through projects to improve the infrastructure. I would add, if you can get someone to pay for it. They talk about inefficient and disorganized international response to hunger, including "excessive food aid without any insistence on guaranteeing sustainability." Maybe some places get excessive food aid but it sounds like many others don't.

The authors suggest support of local and regional farming would be good. I would say that if poor people have no money the local and regional farmers probably won't be eager to give them food for free. What you have to do is figure out ways for people to earn money or get money so they can buy food. That requires conscious efforts by the governments of Africa to make jobs available, to stimulate the economies of the area, and efforts by the governments and banks of developed countries to forgive debts made by these countries by rulers who borrowed huge sums of money and left office with their countries in deep debt to western bankers. Then these bankers insist on getting paid back and western financial institutions inflict "structural adjustments" on the countries. After that, all social programs, such as education, health care, and jobs programs are drastically cut if not ended, so the money saved can be paid back to already rich western bankers. When leaders of developing countries default on their loans they have to worry about being overthrown by U.S. or other western intelligence agents. Maybe it's easier for some leaders to sleep at night if they do what the bankers tell them.

As you can see, these kinds of problems are unlikely to end soon. The authors mention that structural adjustments create "large human development deficits, especially among the poor, and skewed allocation of national revenue and foreign aid so that agriculture and nutrition are neglected." There's probably a lot of malaria that's preventable, but don't hold your breath for bankers to become less greedy in the near future. When it comes to malaria, vaccines are way overdue.

The author of the next article is interested in weeds as food in Africa, especially somewhere in Zimbabwe, where they conducted "semi-structured" interviews. The semi-structure seems like the way to go for interviews; have some questions ready but feel free to let the conversation depart from the questions a bit. If people have something to say that you aren't asking about they might be turning you on to some interesting stuff. The author quotes a couple other studies that find that weeds are important parts of the diets in other parts of Africa (59). My wife and I eat weeds when they're growing in our yard and big enough to pick, especially dandelions. We also have lambs quarter, violets, and thistles. We haven't eaten any thistles but I hear they're edible if you boil them. There's plenty of thistles in the parks around here. Most of our neighbors dump chemicals on their yards in order to have "perfect" grass. I don't want to eat weeds with chemicals, although I eat non-organic vegetables all the time. It would probably be good for us to switch to all organic for our own sakes and to not support the use of chemicals on crops economically.

The author says, "agricultural weeds constitute an important component of farmer's diets around the world." Of course not all weeds are completely edible. There's undoubtedly some that will make you sick or even kill you. The above-mentioned lambs quarter is high in oxalates, which might lead to kidney stones if you go nuts eating lambs quarter. The author found what might be a demographic snapshot of sub-Saharan Africa: 66% of those interviewed were educated "up to primary level". He doesn't say if this means they go up to 6th or 8th grade or what. He says 12.2% were illiterate, which is still too high, but 87.8% literacy isn't bad. Nevertheless, 85% were unemployed living on less than $100 a month. If you're making $100 a month there's very little money for medicine. If your child gets sick there is definitely economic pressure to just wait it out, forgo the drugs. This is where vaccines would save lives. But once again, you have to figure out who's going to pay for the vaccines, because the people who need them most can't afford them.

The author says the main use for edible weeds is leafy vegetables made into relish for porridges of maize, millet, or sorghum, then they boil them with salt and fry them in oil with stuff like tomatoes and onions. It's no doubt tasty and some nutrients probably survive the double cooking. Even so, the author says that weeds are under-used as food in sub-Saharan Africa, which is probably true considering how nutritious some of them are and how little money many Africans have to survive on. Maybe one of the courses in primary schools everywhere should be the choice and preparation of edible weeds, along with facts about nutrition. Nutrient-rich weeds might keep some people from dying of malaria, by bolstering the immune system. Make no mistake, weeds can be quite nutritious. Dandelions are loaded with vitamin A and also have respectable amounts of vitamin C and many other micro-nutrients.

The authors of the next article are curious about vitamin A deficiency, especially in southern Ethiopia. They say vitamin A is important for vision, immunity, epithelial integrity, cellular differentiation, growth and development (60). You surely noticed immunity in there, which is important if you are to fight off malaria and eventually acquire a degree of immunity from it. The authors say that pre-school children and pregnant women suffer most from vitamin A deficiency (VAD). Wow! Another amazing coincidence! Those are the same people most at risk for severe and deadly malaria. I'm not saying that VAD is causing all the deaths from malaria, but maybe some. On the other hand, you might remember that I speculated that Duffy receptor loss, which affects many Africans, that appears to limit the immune activities of platelets, might help people survive malaria. If this is true, it doesn't mean you want to shut down the whole immune response to malaria, just the part that increases the clogging of blood vessels in cerebral and severe malaria. So vitamin A still might be a benefit to someone trying to fight off the disease. I suspect it would be.

The authors say that VAD tends to be higher among women with no education and those "devoid of self-income." Once again we are talking about social problems that should be dealt with by the government: making sure that people are educated, and providing an economy where people can find jobs that pay decent salaries. It seems that governments in Africa have difficulty doing these things and it probably contributes to deaths from malaria. Ignorance of what to do to avoid malaria and what to do once you get it and inability to afford medicine to treat it could all lead to deaths by malaria. The developed industrialized and post-industrial countries that dictate economic terms to less rich countries are just as much to blame as national governments in Africa.

The authors found that 37.9% of the people they tested had VAD. That's a large number, especially considering that you can often get vitamin A from weeds. There's a good chance you wouldn't even have to pay for it. Of course some people don't eat green things because they don't like the taste of them. In cases like that you can't just blame the governments and bankers. We need someone to say, "Hey! Eat 'em anyway!" Maybe Michelle Obama needs to go on a world tour. More power to her for trying to get people to eat good food instead of corporate processed garbage.

The authors figure that if they'd done their surveys in the dry months of May, June and July they'd have found even more VAD. So it seems some people are eating weeds in Ethiopia. Nevertheless, the authors found that maternal night blindness is more common in rural Ethiopia than in urban areas. Out in the country you'd figure there would be plenty of vitamin A rich weeds. But maybe not in the dry months, or maybe people don't know they'd be good to eat and they don't buy vegetables in the store or market. It's questionable whether a vaccine that works for well nourished people will work for malnourished people. The immune system needs certain molecules to work.

The authors of the next article say that not only do 3.5 million mothers and children under 5 die needlessly every year due mostly to under-nutrition, but millions more are permanently disabled mentally and/or physically

(61). It seems likely that malaria could be worse for those who are under nourished. These authors did surveys in Nigeria and found that 6.7% of mothers were under-nourished. They say other researchers have found 25% of Ethiopian women, 43.7% for women in Bangladesh, and 60% for Indian women. Malaria kills people in Bangladesh and India, but my understanding is that it's much worse in Africa. Maybe nutrition status isn't such a good predictor of severity of malaria.

Some researchers from the 1960s and earlier figured malnutrition helped you survive malaria. If part of what kills you when you have malaria is the immune system inadvertently helping to clog small blood vessels as it tries to kill the zillions of parasites in your blood, maybe they're right in some cases. A weak immune response might lead to high parasite loads with relatively few symptoms, if the immune system is responsible for some clogging of blood vessels. A period of few symptoms might give the immune system, what there is of it that works, a chance to make some antibodies, or at least get a bead on what kind of antibodies to make if the building materials for those antibodies ever become available. On the other hand, malnutrition might just delay the blood vessel clogging effects of the immune system until the person gets some food. The best strategy is to give the person's specific immune system a head start on the disease by exposing it to a number of malarial proteins through vaccines. Once again, it probably won't completely prevent the disease, but it will probably make it less deadly and less likely to cause permanent disability.

Vitamin A and zinc supplementation are excellent ways to combat malaria says A.H. Shankar in a recent review (62). Recent field trials have shown this, as well as earlier studies on rats, mice, and ducks, he says. If you're low on vitamin A they might soon be lowering you into the ground if you get malaria. In a recent study of preschool kids in Papua New Guinea cited by Shankar the authors found that vitamin A supplementation cut new cases of malaria by 30% and those who took the vitamin A but still got malaria had 36% lower parasite density. Kids from 12-36 months benefited most with 35% fewer cases and a 68% reduction in parasite density. There doesn't seem to be any dispute, vitamin A helps your immune system fight malaria.

Supplementation is a good cheap way to do it, but there's always a price tag on bottles of vitamins and of course you also have to get the word out. While you're at it, tell them to eat some weeds, dandelions, if they have them, if they want to save some money and a trip to the store. But dandelions contain vitamin E also, which might help malaria parasites, which you don't want to do if you've got malaria. So maybe in this case supplements would be better than the natural source, although there' not a lot of vitamin E in dandelions and there is a lot of vitamin A.

Zinc is right up there with vitamin A in terms of anti-malarial activity, says Shankar. It seems to be a great way to keep parasitemia much lower than it would have been. A study from New Guinea found zinc supplementation resulted in a 69% reduction in cases with high parasitemia, as well as a 38% reduction in number of malaria related health center visits. He quotes a few other studies that help make a strong case for daily zinc supplementation for everyone who lives in the tropics or subtropics or who even occasionally thinks about the tropics.

To summarize Shankar's summaries it seems that iron doesn't have much effect on the disease, and folate might help a little, while vitamins E and C are antioxidants that reduce the immune system's parasite destroying capabilities because the immune system uses oxidation to kill parasites. The several studies that Shankar quotes concerning vitamin E are good reason to avoid it if you get malaria. The less vitamin E you have over the minimum needed for survival when you get malaria, the better.

Shankar says that nutrition with respect to malaria is a complicated subject. Some studies in the distant past that Shankar cites concluded that malnutrition was a good way to combat the disease, but he states that it's accepted now that "general malnutrition is in fact an important risk factor for increased malaria morbidity and mortality." Unfortunately, there are high levels of malnutrition in tropical parts of the world. Some of this needs to be remedied through more equitable wealth distribution. Education might also help many people avoid malnutrition. On the other hand, there will always be those who don't use their money in the best interest of their children. This is where a good vaccine or two might help.

Another recent study investigated antioxidant status of 273 children 1-10 years old who had malaria in Uganda. They found that high plasma concentrations of alpha carotene and lycopene when they showed up at the hospital were associated with early clearance of parasitemia (63). That's a good thing. Get rid of those parasites fast. Alpha carotene is a precursor of vitamin A which the body can convert to vitamin A easily. Lycopene is found in tomatoes, but you can get supplements too if you want, at least here in the U.S., maybe not in sub-Saharan Africa. The authors were especially excited about lycopene. They cited another study that found that tomato consumption is associated with low risk of death by children in Sudan. Maybe the famine relief organizations should make a point of sending many cans of tomato products, as well as tomato seeds, to places. I'm fond of crushed tomatoes. They taste great on a slab of bread. The authors say that low concentrations of vitamin E did not help kids clear the parasites any faster. So maybe vitamin E with malaria isn't so bad after all. I'd still avoid it, especially supplements, if I were in a malaria zone. One of the authors of this article is the author of the previous article, A.H. Shankar. Good work, A.H.!

In addition to vitamins and minerals, one should consider fatty acids' effects on malaria. A recent article states that "Long chain polyunsaturated fatty acids derived from essential fatty acids have been shown to be toxic to Plasmodium falciparum both in vitro and in vivo (64)." So maybe if you get more of these fatty acids in your diet you'd have a better chance of avoiding severe malaria. Sounds like the authors are mostly talking about omega-3 fatty acids.

Looking at the graph the authors of the next article provide shows that omega-3 fatty acids are highest on their list of plasmodial growth inhibition (65). An omega-6 is close behind and an omega-9 and a saturated fatty acid have relatively little effect. Docosahexanoic acid (DHA) is the best, clearly in first place. This you can get from fish oil, but all animals make the stuff. We make it, but not in large quantities, like fish do, the amount we make depends a lot on our diet. If you eat more plant derived omega-3 oils it gives your body the raw materials to make its own DHA. That's the route for me. Someone I know well in Baltimore tells me that in that area they are making what had been plentiful types of fish locally extinct because they net huge numbers of them to make fish oil. They don't make money on the rest of the fish's body, just the oil. Leave the fish alone and figure out a way to synthesize DHA. In the meantime eat flax, which has shorter-chain omega-3 fatty acids that your body can use to maximize DHA production.

Even though the essential fatty acids, the omega-3s, work the best against malaria, fatty acids in general have malaria fighting qualities. Maybe a lot of children in developing countries have low-fat diets. Maybe low everything diets in many cases. The authors say that antioxidants such as vitamin E "markedly reduce the antimalarial activity of the fatty acids". Toward the end of the article the authors say that fish oil had relatively low antimalarial activity, despite relatively large quantities of DHA. The authors figure some of the other fatty acids in fish oil might have interfered somehow, or something like that. Go with the plant derived omega-3s.

The next group of authors took around 200 school kids, ages 9-12, and gave half of them 6 fish oil capsules a day. They looked for behavioral differences between the groups and found none (66). But they did find that the group that took the fish oil capsules, which were rich in

DHA, were much healthier. It looks like they had 60% fewer sick days at school than the group that didn't get the fish oil capsules. That's a big difference. The authors speculate that it was maybe due to less severe cases of malaria thanks to the fish oil. They mention studies done on mice with menhaden fish oil in which the mice were protected by the oil from the ravages of mouse malaria. They add that both oil with and without vitamin E protected the mice. Hopefully after those experiments the surviving mice were released into a big barn full of grain out in the country where they could retire in well-fed luxury as thanks for their contributions to science, and not too many barn owls would be around.

The authors of the next not too recent article say that they have been able to control a number of different drug resistant varieties of malaria by giving the suffering mouse menhaden fish oil and making the rest of their diet deficient in vitamin E (67). It's hard to tell exactly or even vaguely how much menhaden oil they're talking about. But who knows, maybe it would work. The main problem I see is a limited supply of fish oil, that there's probably more malaria sufferers in the world than menhaden fish. The authors say cod liver, anchovy, and salmon oils work well too. Then, as almost an afterthought, they mention that flax oil also showed action against malaria when given in a low vitamin E diet. This is the more practical solution. If all the malaria suffering humans in the world were to start eating fish oil capsules it would cause a mass fish extinction. Plus, it's a rotten way to treat a fish. Let fish have their lives. Go for the plant-derived omega-3s.

The authors of a more recent article say that if you want to use plant-derived omega-3 oils to reduce platelet adhesiveness don't use the oils themselves. They should be taken with the rest of the grains they came in, because otherwise they're missing phosphatides, which are apparently crucial for making omega-3 plant oils reduce platelet adhesiveness. Platelet adhesiveness is possibly part of what causes some cases of malaria to become severe or fatal, if the platelets clog microvessels. On the

94

other hand, the previous group of authors didn't say anything about whole grains rather than refined omega-3 oils being effective against malaria. I'd be inclined to go for the whole grains if I had malaria. But flax grain does have some vitamin E, which might make the malaria worse. Maybe the oil is the way to go. Flip a coin. Complain to your doctors, government officials, and local hot-shot science guys that there isn't at least one vaccine available for malaria yet. It's taken way too long already.

Another way to keep the blood moving is heat, according to the next group of authors. They say that 60°C sauna treatment a couple times a week for 15 minutes each time improved cardiac function in patients with congestive heart failure (68). Clinical symptoms were generally improved including increased peripheral blood flow. The authors figure it was increased nitric oxide (NO) that caused the good results. A high fever for malaria might be helping keep blood vessels from clogging in some cases, although 60°C, which is 140°F, is way higher than the highest fevers. One wonders what a person's body temperature is after they get out of 15 minutes at 140°F. Maybe those temperatures would even kill some parasites. But that's not what the authors were looking at. They found that sauna raised levels of NO which improved vascular endothelial function. There are probably easier ways to raise NO levels, although sauna sounds like it would feel good, as I sit here in Chicago in mid October with the thermostat turned down to save a few bucks.

The title of the next article says that NO given to mice suffering from mouse malaria "decreases brain vascular inflammation, leakage and vascular resistance (69)." That last part about vascular resistance means the blood is flowing better, which means fewer clogged blood vessels. That's great! Hopefully it would work for humans too. The authors used an NO donor called dipropylenetrianineNONOate which they abbreviate "DPTA-NO". The authors say "Murine cerebral malaria (CM) is associated with low NO bioavailability due largely to NO-scavenging by plasma hemoglobin, and exogenous supplementation of NO to PbA-infected mice largely prevents CM." PbA is the kind of mouse malaria they worked with. Of course mice might react differently to NO than humans and maybe their malaria isn't quite the same. But still, this suggests that NO might help some sufferers of human CM. The authors go on to say that exogenous NO "attenuated" but did not prevent brain vascular inflammation in mice in their latest study. If you find a way to attenuate CM in humans it could save lives, depending on how much attenuation you get. The authors injected DPTA-NO into the mice. So DPTA-NO looks like something you might get at a hospital. If you're not close to a hospital or clinic or feel that you can't afford to go to one or to a doctor you might miss out on a treatment like DPTA-NO.

 The authors of another recent study used nitorglycerine, the same stuff heart patients often use on their own when they get chest pains. Nitroglycerine is an NO donor that raises NO levels in blood vessels. The authors put it on the skin of mice with cerebral malaria (CM). They found that the nitroglycerine dramatically increased the survival of their CM afflicted mice (70). It brought mortality down from 67% to 11% when used by itself. The authors call the chemical they used glyceryl trinitrate, but it's also known as nitroglycerine. Every drug store here in the U.S. probably has it. It wouldn't be hard to make available in Africa, somewhat available at least. You could probably inhale it and get good results too. But then again, there will be people who don't want to pay for the drug or who can't pay or who don't want to travel all the way to the nearest drug store or who misjudge the severity of the disease and as a result people die or suffer brain damage. That's why vaccines are the way to go. You can get some protection from malaria at a time when you're not miserably sick, just about any time, in fact. You don't have to be able to recognize cerebral malaria. Keep in mind malaria is one of many tropical diseases. They're not all easy to tell apart from one another. A vaccine, you get it at a time that's convenient for you, preferably not too early in life. Give the kid's immune system time to mature. But then give her the vaccine.

Education and Malaria

This next section is about education especially concerning malaria, in Africa. Lots of people die of malaria in other countries too, but Africa seems hardest hit, and education might have something to do with that. A study from the West African Journal of Medicine surveyed 376 mothers and care givers of kids under 5 about their knowledge and practices concerning malaria. Less than half of them knew how malaria was transmitted, 46.8% (71). That's pretty sad. You can bet few of the 53% of people surveyed who don't know about the mosquito-malaria connection will be using bed nets.

81% used Tylenol for malaria. Another 21.5% used chlorquine, which might actually help, but many cases of malaria are resistant to it now. 25.5% of mothers and care givers gave the youngsters "agbo", which is sold on the street. The ingredients of agbo can vary. A website I found says they are "leaves, chemicals, gin". Some people in Nigeria lover agbo and defend it vigorously online. Others say the ingredients can destroy your liver and kidneys. I suppose it depends on the types of leaves and chemicals your agbo maker uses. I used to like putting parsley in the blender and making a parsley drink. It tastes good and I thought it was healthy, but I found out parsley is sky-high in oxalates, which are thought to help cause kidney stones. But a parsley blend-up every now and then probably won't hurt you. Maybe agbo's the same way in some cases.

Only 4.3% of the kids got an anti-malarial the day the illness began. On the one hand you might say, "Who knows exactly what this disease is? Why waste good medicine if it's not malaria?" On the other hand, knowing malaria is a killer, why take chances? Give the kid the anti-malarial just in case. The latter practice is best. This article was written in 2001, when artemisinin-containing drugs had not been on the market long, which probably accounts for the fact that nobody mentioned the stuff at all. Hopefully, since then west Africans have become more knowledgeable about malaria, but there's probably still a large percentage that know very little.

Another article from around that time tells about education in general in sub-Saharan Africa. The authors looked at seven countries to find determinants of school enrollment and completion of fourth grade. They say that in those countries "a substantial majority" of 10-14 year olds were enrolled in school (72). Unfortunately "many fewer" children by that age had gotten past the fourth grade level. I don't know what the actually numbers are because they want me to pay a big pile of bucks for this article and I won't do it, but I think we get the idea. The education systems in these countries could be better. The authors say that if your parents are well-educated and /or they're doing well financially you stand a better chance of being in school and doing well there. They also say that in households headed by females the kids tended to get better educations. Maybe a father isn't that great of a thing to have in some cases, apart from the sperm donation. If the old pops gets overly attached to the agbo, it could cause problems.

Here's an article that looks at HIV with respect to education. They find that the better educated you are, the better the chance you'll avoid HIV (73). But before 1996 it was the opposite say the authors. Back then having an education probably helped you to be more appealing as a sex partner and the facts about HIV weren't well known in sub-Saharan Africa. It switched in '96. That's when educated people, who in most cases could probably read, found out about the dangers of HIV more than the uneducated. The authors argument: increased education levels are "urgently needed." My guess is that this would save lives that would otherwise be lost to malaria also. The authors say that one of the best things you can do to increase school enrollment is to eliminate fees for grade school. Make education free. If you have to pay for it lots of people won't go. Give the kids K-12 free of charge, or better still, give 'em 4 years of college too. Of course education programs cost money, and they're the types of programs most commonly cut when the western bankers come around looking for their loan money, complete with intelligence agencies as enforcers.

This next article shows how little people in Yemen know about malaria. The authors had group discussions and questionnaires about malaria and found that knowledge of malaria transmission was vague (74). It seems that in many cases mothers didn't know mosquitoes were involved. Part of the problem in Yemen is that women have a low rate of literacy, 35%, compared to 69% for men, say the authors. This sexist educational policy definitely leads to unnecessarily high numbers of dead children in that country. The authors emphatically call for better education in Yemen. Many people there think malaria is transmitted by flies according to the authors, who also say that the idea that malaria is transmitted through breast milk is another totally false and potentially deadly idea that is popular in this land of many small coffins.

Bed nets: "rarely used" say the authors. If you don't understand the mosquito-malaria connection I suppose bed nets wouldn't seem crucial, although if you think flies are the carriers you might still opt for the bed nets. On the other hand, the flies we have here in northern Illinois are not active in the dark. They're not nocturnal, like mosquitoes.

The authors say that 78% of parents delay seeking medical treatment for malaria. They add, "Prevention of progression of disease from mild to severe depends on early recognition of symptoms and appropriate action". At some point, hopefully early, you bite the bullet and resolve to spend some money in order to keep your child healthy. The authors say that in Yemen and many African countries women don't have money and have to consult with a husband or male relative to bring the child in or get treatment. This powerlessness of women probably leads to many children's deaths.

The authors quote a study from Uganda that found mothers decided to go for medical treatment only if it was free. If early treatment is important for avoiding severe malaria you can see this practice will lead to children's deaths. The authors urge better education programs in Yemen. That goes for the rest of the world too. And you may as well toss in worldwide universal free health care too, including free antimalarial drugs. At the end of the article the authors say that use of bed nets needs to be highlighted. That's right! They're cheap and effective. Mosquitoes love biting people while they sleep. They're much less likely to get slapped. Then they can fly off and bit some more people.

You would think bed nets would be used a lot in sub-Saharan Africa, but they're not, according to the next article, which quotes studies that say only 2% of children sleep under bed nets (75). Only 2% bed net use for children in sub-Saharan Africa. Wow! That's terrible. You figure they probably don't want their kids to die, so it must be ignorance or lack of ways to get bed nets. The authors looked at child mortality in general in a part of Ethiopia and found that the three main causes of death were pneumonia, diarrhea and malaria, with 29.7%, 23% and 23% respectively. With that much pneumonia you wonder if maybe the kids could use a few blankets on their beds, as well as the nets. Death from diarrhea suggests that they have some bad sources of water in that part of Ethiopia. The authors considered malnutrition a factor in at least 38% of children's deaths, maybe more due to kids they couldn't tell were malnourished just by looking at them. Once again, education and access to money would help here. The authors say that breast feeding and being from a family with fewer than five children and vaccinations all helped children survive according to their study.

The authors say that only 36% of the kids were

fully vaccinated but 70% of them got the BCG vaccine, which is mainly for tuberculosis. But we will see shortly that it also protects against malaria. If you add some malarial antigens to it it will almost certainly give even more antimalarial protection. What they're waiting for on this, nobody knows. But my guess is somebody figures it's not profitable enough.

The authors say that risk of mortality was 6 times higher for kids who weren't vaccinated. That's a very big difference. Vaccines are the way to go and a malaria vaccine or two should be among them. Probably one for Ebola too. I just read that back in 1999 they had a vaccine that kept all the monkeys it was given to from getting Ebola, while those that didn't get the vaccine died. It was 100% effective for monkeys but they never went on to test it for humans because they didn't think Ebola was actually that dangerous. Recently about 10,000 people mostly in west Africa have died from it. One hopes that would be a big enough number for the drug companies to notice. They've been dragging their asses on all kinds of vaccines.

Immunity and Malaria

This next section has more about vaccines and immunity in general with respect to malaria. The authors of the first article say that mixed infections of Plasmodium vivax with Plasmodium falciparum tend to be much less severe (76). You might think two different kinds of malaria at once would be especially deadly, but it's just the opposite. The authors say the mixed infection, P. vivax and P. falciparum "is approximately a quarter as severe as single P. falciparum infection." They say that P. falciparum causes "immunosuppression during the parasitaemic stage." But P. vivax wakes up the suppressed immune system and helps it fight off P. falciparum. The authors say these mixed infections are common in various places of low endemicity for P. falciparum, especially Thailand. So there's plenty of evidence for how these mixed infections are.

The authors say that mixed infections usually have low levels of parasitemia. They suggest that P. vivax activates the killer function of a class of T-cells and the T-cells kill many of the parasites. They also note that P. vivax induces a higher temperature fever that kills more P. falciparum. Maybe the sauna treatment we discussed a while ago for keeping blood moving would have the added attraction of killing more parasites. Up here in Chicago if you want ready access to a sauna you have to join a health club, which costs money. It seems that many people in Africa don't have the money to join a health club. Sauna treatment for P. falciparum malaria might also be a good subject for a study or two, just out of curiosity, because you won't see saunas springing up all over Africa soon.

The authors also suggest putting some P. vivax antigens in with P. falciparum antigens for a vaccine. That's an idea that might work. What seems more likely to work is to give people who have P. falciparum a shot of P. vivax antigens. I'm afraid with the P. vivax antigens in the vaccine the immune system won't see the P. vivax antigens when a person gets P. falciparum malaria so that person won't have the extra immune activation. But maybe it would work. Who knows? Let's give it a try.

The authors of the next article say that the BCG vaccine, which was originally developed to combat tuberculosis, provides other general health benefits to those vaccinated, including protection against asthma, leprosy, and malaria (77). BCG's effectiveness against tuberculosis is from 0-80% say the authors, but they strongly urge governments not to discontinue its use. Even if the BCG vaccine doesn't completely prevent cases of TB, it consistently keeps them from becoming severe, say the authors. So this is obviously a vaccine that is working. Even if it doesn't absolutely prevent TB it keeps it from becoming severe, thus saving lives. At this point a malaria vaccine that performed like this would be excellent and save many lives. This idea that the malaria vaccine has to prevent a high percentage of cases of malaria otherwise it's no good is killing people.

The authors say that the BCG vaccine induces expression of non-specific immune molecules, including "antimicrobial peptides" which help to limit infections of "unrelated pathogens such as Plasmodium parasites." The authors quote a couple studies that found a 45% decrease in infant mortality when the BCG vaccine was used. In a cited study from Brazil there was a 50% reduction in pneumonia related deaths when the BCG vaccine was given. The authors say that the BCG bacteria are often put into the bladder for bladder cancer. They whip up an immune response against cancer too, it seems. The authors say that in animals it was found that the BCG vaccine works against a number of pathogens including those that cause babesia, toxoplasmosis, and Chagas disease, as well as malaria.

The authors note that other vaccines have benefits beyond protection from a single disease. They say that the reduction in mortality caused by the measles vaccine "cannot be solely explained by decreased rates of measles infections." Maybe the measles vaccine helps you fight off malaria too.

BCG protection against human malaria might be very strong. The authors quote a study that found that in mice who were given mouse malaria the ones who got a BCG vaccine first had dramatically lower levels of parasitemia. By 16 days after infection the BCG vaccinated mice had a 93% reduction in parasitemia compared to non-vaccinated mice. That sounds like a big difference.

The authors say that BCG vaccination induces a bunch of immune molecules including "4 antimicrobial compounds, three IL-1 related molecules, and several chemokines." The authors describe the antimicrobial compound lactoferrin. They say it "inhibits the growth of bacteria, viruses and parasites by multiple mechanisms including sequestering iron, destabilizing microbial membranes, and interfering with microbial adherence to host cells." They say it was found to block adherence of mouse malaria parasites to host cells, and it inhibits P. falciparum growth in vitro. The authors say that lactoferrin given as a treatment for malaria significantly reduces parasitemia. Yet there's nothing about lactoferrin that is specific to malaria. It's a good molecule to have when you get just about any disease. You get a bunch of it from the BCG vaccine. The authors say that the BCG vaccine causes 11 immune related genes to be expressed which are normally suppressed by the malaria parasites. One of these genes, Nos2, is a nitric oxide synthase, which makes nitric oxide (NO), which is in short supply with malaria. NO can help keep blood moving in small blood vessels, you recall. In short, the authors are in love with the BCG vaccine and urge its continued use.

BCG is short for Bacillus calmette-guerin. The authors of the next article say that Calmette and Guerin were a bacteriologist and his assistant, respectively, in France in 1908 (78). They say these guys raised bovine tuberculosis bacteria on a glycerin-bile-potato mixture that made the bacteria less virulent after "repeated subculturing". Then they got the idea that maybe it would make a good vaccine. The authors don't say exactly how the two determined if the bacteria were virulent. Hopefully it was done in a fully ethical manner.

The U.S. has never done mass BCG vaccinations, but many other countries have, according to the authors, including France, the UK, the Soviet Union, Brazil, Pakistan, and India. They add that it's a very safe vaccine that's given as an injection intradermally, but if you accidentally go all the way under the skin, "subcutaneously", there can be problems and you might need to take some antibiotics. That sounds like a tricky maneuver, the intradermal injection without going subcutaneous, but apparently if you get people who know what they're doing...

The authors say the BCG vaccine has been used to

boost the immune response to a variety of cancers, including bladder cancer, colorectal cancer, lung cancer, melanoma, and malignant peripheral nerve sheath tumor. These authors also mention that the BCG vaccine's protective effect for tuberculosis is highly variable, 0%-80%. In the UK they say it's 60%-80% but effectiveness seems to drop as you get closer to the equator for some reason. Even so, the authors mention that BCG's greatest effect is at preventing miliary TB and TB meningitis, the worst forms of TB. Miliary TB is TB that's spread throughout the lungs and possibly other organs of the body. Wikipedia says if untreated it's almost always fatal.

So somehow, back 100 years or so ago, the perfectionists lost out and a good vaccine was approved even though it didn't prevent the disease in almost all cases. Yes, the disease is still there sometimes, but it's not as severe. That's a huge benefit.

The authors list a number of possible reasons for the BCG vaccine being less effective at preventing tuberculosis as you get closer to the equator. The most convincing one is concurrent parasitic infection. This has been found to change the immune response to BCG, say the authors. As you get closer to the equator there is less snow and ice to kill parasites and parasite carriers for part of the year, making concurrent infections more likely the closer to the equator you get.

The authors say that to give the BCG vaccine to an immunocompromised person can result in a life-threatening infection. Unfortunately in Africa there are many children carrying the HIV virus, which might make the BCG vaccine less practical there, as well as any other live vaccine. This is why there should be a variety of malaria vaccines available. If a person can't handle a live vaccine, there ought to be alternatives.

A University of California at San Francisco website I just looked at says that vaccinations of any kind might not be a good thing for HIV-positive people since activation of CD4 cells tends to speed up their destruction by HIV. Nevertheless, some researchers still think some vaccinations are good for HIV positive people, according to Wikipedia. So this vaccine idea might be complicated to some extent by HIV. One website says that 1.8% of South African children are HIV positive. Another website says that in 2008 the HIV infection rate for 10 year-olds was 3.2% but was expected to fall to 1.6% by 2020. Nigeria, the most populous country in sub-Saharan Africa, has an overall 3.2% HIV infection rate, which sounds low, but translates to lots of infected children. The National Institutes of Health in the U.S. have a detailed schedule of vaccinations for HIV positive children, which includes a lot of vaccines. If you give HIV positive kids a malaria vaccine, if they ever make them available, it should not be a live vaccine, would be my guess. And make sure the kid is healthy otherwise when you give it to her. You don't want to send her into the final tailspin of death.

A few recent articles suggest that malaria antigens be combined with the BCG vaccine. The first group of authors figure the P. falciparum circumsporozoite protein would be a good one to use with the BCG vaccine as sort of an adjuvant (79). The authors got stronger immune responses with the combination than with just the BCG vaccine when they tried it on mice. This suggests that some of the the increased activation was specific to malaria antigens. My finding over the years is that many people are mouse-like, but there's always a few that aren't, even if you wish they were. The authors grew the circumsporozoite proteins right on the BCG bacteria, which probably prolonged the exposure of the circumporozoited proteins to the immune system, which is a plus.

Another group of authors grew BCG bacteria with a different malarial protein, a chunk of a serine repeat antigen (SERA) found on P. falciparum merozoites (80). That would be the blood stage of the disease, which the authors remind us is the time when the major symptoms of malaria occur. This would be a great time for the immune system to be able to zero in on at least one malarial antigen quickly. It might be the difference between life and death.

106

The authors say the BCG-SERA vaccine produced high levels of specific immunoglobulins when tested in mice, and that the immunoglobulins were reactive to P. falciparum merozoites. The authors say that previous studies found that anti-SERA antibodies can agglutinate malarial merozoites and schizonts and block merozoite dispersal. SERA sounds like a good malaria antigen for the immune system to recognize early. Schizonts are the little malarial beasts found in the liver stage of the disease. May as well kill a bunch of them too if possible.

Another group of authors are enthusiastic about using a recombinant BCG vaccine with the C-terminus of merozoite surface protein-1 (MSP-1C) added to the BCG bacteria (81). The authors say MSP-1C has been extensively studied and it's conserved across all Plasmodium species. Sounds like it might make a great vaccine, that might help fight P. vivax, as well as other types of malaria besides the deadly P. falciparum. The authors say this protein is important for merozoite invasion of red blood cells, and that antibodies to it have been associated with asymptomatic malaria in animals. Sounds like the authors have yet another excellent candidate for a vaccine antigen and an adjuvant that has already been shown to protect against malaria without even having any malarial antigens. Put 'em together and try 'em out. There have been way too many delays and too much waiting for perfection concerning malaria vaccines. Time to roll 'em out and keep 'em coming.

Citations

1. Boffey PM, Malaria Vaccine Is Near, U.S. Health Officials Say. New York Times, August 3, 1984
2. Ross MC, *Dangerous Beauty: Life and Death in Africa: True Stories from a Safari Guide.* Miramax Books, New York City, 2001, 37
3. Ouédraogo A, Tiono AB, Diarra A, Sanon S, Yaro JB, Ouedraogo E, Bougouma EC, Soulama I, Gansané A, Ouedraogo A, Konate AT, Nebie I, Watson NL, Sanza M, Dube TJ, Sirima SB 2013 Malaria morbidity in high and seasonal malaria transmission area of Burkina Faso. PLoS One 8(1)
4. Vliegenthart-Jongbloed K, de Mendonça Melo M, van Wolfswinkel ME, Koelewijn R, van Hellemond JJ, van Genderen PJ 2013 Severity of imported malaria: protective effect of taking malaria chemoprophylaxis. Malaria Journal 12:265
5. Moorthy VS, Hutubessy R, Newman RD, Hombach J 2012 Decision-making on malaria vaccine introduction: the role of cost-effectiveness analyses. Bulletin of the World Health Organization 90(11):864-6
6. Riley EM1, Wagner GE, Akanmori BD, Koram KA 2001 Do maternally acquired antibodies protect infants from malaria infection? Parasite Immunology 23(2):51-9.
7. Jiang L, Gaur D, Mu J, Zhou H, Long CA, Miller LH 2011 Evidence for erythrocyte-binding antigen 175 as a component of a ligand-blocking blood-stage malaria vaccine. Proceedings of the National Academy of Sciences of the United States of America 108(18):7553-8
8. Duffy PE, Sahu T, Akue A, Milman N, Anderson C 2012 Pre-erythrocytic malaria vaccines: identifying the targets. Expert Review of Vaccines 11(10):1261-80.
9. Abdulla S, Oberholzer, Juma O, Kubhoja S,

Machera F, Membi C, Omari S, Urassa A, Mshinda H, Jumanne A, Salim N, Shomari M, Aebi T, Schellenberg DM, Carter T, Villafana T, Demoitié M, Dubois MC, Leach A, Lievens M, Vekemans J, Cohen J, Ballou WR, Tanner M 2008 Safety and Immunogenicity of RTS,S/AS02D Malaria Vaccine in Infants. The New England Journal of Medicine 359:2533-2544

10. Agnandji ST et al. 2011 RTS,S Clinical Trials Partnership 2011 First results of phase 3 trial of RTS,S/AS01 malaria vaccine in African children. New England Journal of Medicine 365(20):1863-75

11. Warimwe GM, Recker M, Kiragu EW, Buckee CO, Wambua J, Musyoki JN, Marsh K, Bull PC mail 2013 Plasmodium falciparum var gene expression homogeneity as a marker of the host-parasite relationship under different levels of naturally acquired immunity to malaria. PLOS One

12. Chuangchaiya S, Persson KER 2013 How should antibodies against P. falciparum merozoite antigens be measured? Journal of Tropical Medicine

13. Segeja MD, Mmbando BP, Seth MD, Lusingu JP, Lemnge MM 2010 Acquisition of antibodies to merozoite surface protein 3 among residents of Korogwe, north eastern Tanzania. BMC Infectious Diseases 10:55

14. Richards JS, Arumugam TU, Reiling L, Healer J, Hodder AN, Fowkes FJ, Cross N, Langer C, Takeo S, Uboldi AD, Thompson JK, Gilson PR, Coppel RL, Siba PM, King CL, Torii M, Chitnis CE, Narum DL, Mueller I, Crabb BS, Cowman AF, Tsuboi T, Beeson JG 2013 Identification and prioritization of merozoite antigens as targets of protective human immunity to Plasmodium falciparum malaria for vaccine and biomarker development. Journal of Immunology 191(2):795-

809
15. Vaughan AM, Wang R, Kappe SH 2010 Genetically engineered, attenuated whole-cell vaccine approaches for malaria. Human Vaccines 6(1):107-13
16. VanBuskirk KM1, O'Neill MT, De La Vega P, Maier AG, Krzych U, Williams J, Dowler MG, Sacci JB Jr, Kangwanrangsan N, Tsuboi T, Kneteman NM, Heppner DG Jr, Murdock BA, Mikolajczak SA, Aly AS, Cowman AF, Kappe SH 2009 Preerythrocytic, live-attenuated Plasmodium falciparum vaccine candidates by design. Proceedings of the National Academy of Sciences of the United States of America 106(31):13004-9
17. Nussenzweig RS, Long CA 1994 Malaria vaccines: multiple targets. Science 265(5177):1381-3
18. Febir LG, Asante KP, Dzorgbo DB, Senah KA, Letsa TS, Owusu-Agyei S 2013 Community perceptions of a malaria vaccine in the Kintampo districts of Ghana. Malaria Journal 12:156
19. Hill AV, Reyes-Sandoval A, O'Hara G, Ewer K, Lawrie A, Goodman A, Nicosia A, Folgori A, Colloca S, Cortese R, Gilbert SC, Draper SJ 2010 Prime-boost vectored malaria vaccines: progress and prospects. Human Vaccines 6(1):78-83
20. Murhandarwati EE, Wang L, de Silva HD, Ma C, Plebanski M, Black CG, Coppel RL 2010 Growth-inhibitory antibodies are not necessary for protective immunity to malaria infection. Infection and Immunity 78(2):680-7
21. Othoro C, Johnston D, Lee R, Soverow J, Bystryn JC, Nardin E 2008 Enhanced immunogenicity of Plasmodium falciparum peptide vaccines using a topical adjuvant containing a potent synthetic Toll-like receptor 7 agonist, imiquimod. Infection and Immunity 77(2):739-48
22. Noone C, Parkinson M, Dowling DJ, Aldridge A, Kirwan P, Molloy SF, Asaolu SO, Holland C,

O'Neill SM 2013 Plasma cytokines, chemokines and cellular immune responses in pre-school Nigerian children infected with Plasmodium falciparum. Malaria Journal 12:5

23. Fernandez-Arias C, Lopez JP, Hernandez-Perez JN, Bautista-Ojeda MD, Branch O, Rodriguez A 2013 Malaria inhibits surface expression of complement receptor 1 in monocytes/macrophages, causing decreased immune complex internalization. Journal of Immunology 190(7):3363-72

24. Pradhan V, Ghosh K 2012 Immunological disturbances associated with malarial infection. Journal of Parasitic Diseases 37(1):11-5

25. Carlson J, Nash GB, Gabutti V, al-Yaman F, Wahlgren M 1994 Natural protection against severe Plasmodium falciparum malaria due to impaired rosette formation. Blood 84(11):3909-14

26. Verra F, Simpore J, Warimwe GM, Tetteh KK, Howard T, Osier FHA, Bancone G, Avellino P, Blot I, Fegan G, Bull PC, Williams TN, Conway DJ, Marsh K, Modiano D 2007 Haemoglobin C and S Role in Acquired Immunity against Plasmodium falciparum Malaria. PLOS One

27. Rowe JA1, Claessens A, Corrigan RA, Arman M 2009 Adhesion of Plasmodium falciparum-infected erythrocytes to human cells: molecular mechanisms and therapeutic implications. Expert Reviews in Molecular Medicine 26:11

28. Tembo DL, Montgomery J, Craig AG, Wassmer SC 2013 A simple protocol for platelet-mediated clumping of Plasmodium falciparum-infected erythrocytes in a resource poor setting. Journal of Visualized Experiments

29. Arman M, Raza A, Tempest LJ, Lyke KE, Thera MA, Koné A, Plowe CV, Doumbo OK, Rowe JA 2007 Platelet-mediated clumping of Plasmodium falciparum infected erythrocytes is associated with high parasitemia but not severe clinical

manifestations of malaria in African children. American Journal of Tropical Medicine and Hygiene 77(5):943-6

30. Leitgeb AM, Blomqvist K, Cho-Ngwa F, Samje M, Nde P, Titanji V, Wahlgren M 2011 Low anticoagulant heparin disrupts Plasmodium falciparum rosettes in fresh clinical isolates. American Journal of Tropical Medicine and Hygiene 84(3):390-6

31. Gandhi M 2007 Complement receptor 1 and the molecular pathogenesis of malaria. Indian Journal of Human Genetics 13(2):39–47

32. Tham WH, Wilson DW, Lopaticki S, Schmidt CQ, Tetteh-Quarcoo PB, Barlow PN, Richard D, Corbin JE, Beeson JG, Cowman AF 2010 Complement receptor 1 is the host erythrocyte receptor for Plasmodium falciparum PfRh4 invasion ligand. Proceedings of the National Academy of Sciences of the United States of America 107(40):17327-32

33. Juillerat A1, Lewit-Bentley A, Guillotte M, Gangnard S, Hessel A, Baron B, Vigan-Womas I, England P, Mercereau-Puijalon O, Bentley GA 2011 Structure of a Plasmodium falciparum PfEMP1 rosetting domain reveals a role for the N-terminal segment in heparin-mediated rosette inhibition. Proceedings of the National Academy of Sciences of the United States of America 108(13):5243-8

34. Ghumra A, Semblat JP, Ataide R, Kifude C, Adams Y, Claessens A, Anong DN, Bull PC, Fennell C, Arman M, Amambua-Ngwa A, Walther M, Conway DJ, Kassambara L, Doumbo OK, Raza A, Rowe JA 2012 Induction of strain-transcending antibodies against Group A PfEMP1 surface antigens from virulent malaria parasites. PLoS Pathogens 8(4)

35. Angeletti D, Albrecht L, Wahlgren M, Moll K 2013 Analysis of antibody induction upon

immunization with distinct NTS-DBL1α-domains of PfEMP1 from rosetting Plasmodium falciparum parasites. Malaria Journal 12:32

36. Ghumra A, Khunrae P, Ataide R, Raza A, Rogerson SJ, Higgins MK, Rowe JA 2011 Immunisation with recombinant PfEMP1 domains elicits functional rosette-inhibiting and phagocytosis-inducing antibodies to Plasmodium falciparum. PLoS One 6(1)

37. Cockburn IA, Mackinnon MJ, O'Donnell A, Allen SJ, Moulds JM, Baisor M, Bockarie M, Reeder JC, Rowe JA 2004 A human complement receptor 1 polymorphism that reduces Plasmodium falciparum rosetting confers protection against severe malaria. Proceedings of the National Academy of Sciences of the United States of America 101(1):272-7

38. EP Vichinsky 2014 Sickle cell trait. Uptodate.com

39. Shin W, Yoon J, Oh GT, Ryoo S 2013 Korean red ginseng inhibits arginase and contributes to endotheliumdependent vasorelaxation through endothelial nitric oxide synthase coupling. Journal of Ginseng Research 37(1):64-73

40. Lei C, Yu B, Shahid M, Beloiartsev A, Bloch KD, Zapol WM 2012 Inhaled nitric oxide attenuates the adverse effects of transfusing stored syngeneic erythrocytes in mice with endothelial dysfunction after hemorrhagic shock. Anesthesiology 117(6):1190-202

41. Hendgen-Cotta UB, Luedike P, Totzeck M, Kropp M, Schicho A, Stock P, Rammos C, Niessen M, Heiss C, Lundberg JO, Weitzberg E, Kelm M, Rassaf T 2012 Dietary nitrate supplementation improves revascularization in chronic ischemia. Circulation 126(16):1983-92

42. YC Martins, GM Zanini, JA Frangos, LJM Carvalho 2012 Efficacy of different nitric oxide-based strategies in preventing experimental cerebral malaria by Plasmodium berghei ANKA.

PloS one
43. McMorran BJ, Burgio G, Foote SJ 2013 New insights into the protective power of platelets in malaria infection. Communicative & Integrative Biology 1;6(3)
44. Cook SP 2013 The quest for affordable artemisinin. Future Medicinal Chemisty 5(3):233-6
45. Antoine T, Fisher N, Amewu R, O'Neill PM, Ward SA, Biagini GA 2014 Rapid kill of malaria parasites by artemisinin and semi-synthetic endoperoxides involves ROS-dependent depolarization of the membrane potential. Journal of Antimicrobial Chemotherapy 69(4)
46. Newton PN, Green MD, Mildenhall DC, Plançon A, Nettey H, Nyadong L, Hostetler DM, Swamidoss I, Harris GA, Powell K, Timmermans AE, Amin AA, Opuni SK, Barbereau S, Faurant C, Soong RC, Faure K, Thevanayagam J, Fernandes P, Kaur H, Angus B, Stepniewska K, Guerin PJ, Fernández FM 2011 Poor quality vital anti-malarials in Africa - an urgent neglected public health priority. Malaria Journal
47. Ioset JR, Kaur H 2009 Simple Field Assays to Check Quality of Current Artemisinin-Based Antimalarial Combination Formulations. Plos One
48. Atemnkeng MA, De Cock K, Plaizier-Vercammen J 2007 Quality control of active ingredients in artemisinin-derivative antimalarials within Kenya and DR Congo. Tropical Medicine and International Health 12(1):68-74
49. Ambroise-Thomas P 2012 The tragedy caused by fake antimalarial drugs. Mediterranean Journal of Hematology and Infectious Diseases 4(1)
50. Almuzaini T, Choonara I, Sammons H 2013 Substandard and counterfeit medicines: a systematic review of the literature. BMJ Open 3(8)
51. Kalanda BF, Verhoeff FH, Brabin BJ 2006 Breast and complementary feeding practices in relation to

114

morbidity and growth in Malawian infants. European Journal of Clinical Nutrition 60(3):401-7

52. Safeukui-Noubissi I, Ranque S, Poudiougou B, Keita M, Traoré A, Traoré D, Diakité M, Cissé MB, Keita MM, Dessein A, Doumbo OK 2004 Risk factors for severe malaria in Bamako, Mali: a matched case-control study. Microbes and Infection 6(6):572-8

53. Kassim OO, Ako-Anai KA, Torimiro SE, Hollowell GP, Okoye VC, Martin SK 2000 Inhibitory factors in breastmilk, maternal and infant sera against in vitro growth of Plasmodium falciparum malaria parasite. Journal of Tropical Pediatrics 46(2):92-6

54. Sawatzki G 1997 Lactoferrin in Infant Formulas. Experimental Biology and Medicine 28:389-397

55. Chirico G, Marzollo R, Cortinovis S, Fonte C, Gasparoni A 2008 Antiinfective properties of human milk. The Journal of Nutrition 138(9):1801S-1806S

56. Yang S 2007 HIV in breastmilk killed by flash-heating, new study finds. UC Berkley News, May 21

57. Fonseca MJ, Moreira A, Moreira P, Delgado L, Teixeira V, Padrão P 2010 Duration of breastfeeding and the risk of childhood asthma in children living in urban areas. Journal of Investigative Allergology and Clinical Immunology 20(4):357-8

58. Lartey A 2008 Maternal and child nutrition in Sub-Saharan Africa: challenges and interventions. The Proceedings of the Nutrition Society 67(1):105-8

59. Bain LE, Awah PK, Geraldine N, Kindong NP, Sigal Y, Bernard N, Tanjeko AT 2013 Malnutrition in Sub – Saharan Africa: burden, causes and prospects. The Pan African Medical Journal 15:120

60. Maroyi A 2013 Use of weeds as traditional

vegetables in Shurugwi District, Zimbabwe. Journal of Ethnobiology and Ethnomedicine 9:60

61. Gebreselassie SG, Gase FE, Deressa MU 2013 Prevalence and correlates of prenatal vitamin A deficiency in rural Sidama, Southern Ethiopia. Journal of Health, Population, and Nutrition 31(2):185-94

62. Senbanjo IO, Olayiwola IO, Afolabi WA, Senbanjo OC 2013 Maternal and child under-nutrition in rural and urban communities of Lagos state, Nigeria: the relationship and risk factors. BMC Research Notes 6:286

63. Shankar AH 2000 Nutritional modulation of malaria morbidity and mortality. The Journal of Infectious Diseases.182 Suppl 1:S37-53.

64. Metzger A, Mukasa G, Shankar AH, Ndeezi G, Melikian G, Semba RD 2001 Antioxidant status and acute malaria in children in Kampala, Uganda. The American Journal of Tropical Medecine and Hygiene 65(2):115-9

65. Arun Kumar C, Das UN 1999 Lipid peroxides, nitric oxide and essential fatty acids in patients with Plasmodium falciparum malaria. Prostaglandins, Leukotreines, and Essential Fatty Acids 61(4):255-8.

66. Kumaratilake LM, Robinson BS, Ferrante A, Poulos A 1992 Antimalarial properties of n-3 and n-6 polyunsaturated fatty acids: in vitro effects on Plasmodium falciparum and in vivo effects on P. berghei. The Journal of Clinical Investigations 89(3):961-7

67. Hamazaki K, Syafruddin D, Tunru IS, Azwir MF, Asih PB, Sawazaki S, Hamazaki T 2008 The effects of docosahexaenoic acid-rich fish oil on behavior, school attendance rate and malaria infection in school children--a double-blind, randomized, placebo-controlled trial in Lampung, Indonesia. Asia Pacific Journal of Clinical Nutrition 17(2):258-63

68. Levander OA, Ager AL Jr, Morris VC, May RG 1989 Menhaden-fish oil in a vitamin E-deficient diet: protection against chloroquine-resistant malaria in mice. The American Journal of Clinical Nutrition 50(6):1237-9

69. Kihara T, Biro S, Imamura M, Yoshifuku S, Takasaki K, Ikeda Y, Otuji Y, Minagoe S, Toyama Y, Tei C 2002 Repeated sauna treatment improves vascular endothelial and cardiac function in patients with chronic heart failure. Journal of the American College of Cardiology 39(5):754-9

70. Zanini GM, Cabrales P, Barkho W, Frangos JA, Carvalho LJ 2011 Exogenous nitric oxide decreases brain vascular inflammation, leakage and venular resistance during Plasmodium berghei ANKA infection in mice. Journal of Neuroinflammation 8:66

71. Orjuela-Sánchez P, Ong PK, Zanini GM, Melchior B, Martins YC, Meays D, Frangos JA, Carvalho LJ 2013 Transdermal glyceryl trinitrate as an effective adjunctive treatment with artemether for late-stage experimental cerebral malaria. Antimicrobial Agents and Chemotherapy 57(11):5462-71

72. Fawole OI, Onadeko MO 2001 Knowledge and home management of malaria fever by mothers and care givers of under five children. West African Journal of Medicine 20(2):152-7

73. Lloyd CB, Blanc AK 1996 Children's schooling in sub-Saharan Africa: the role of fathers, mothers, and others. Population and Development Review 22(2):265-298

74. Hargreaves JR, Bonell CP, Boler T, Boccia D, Birdthistle I, Fletcher A, Pronyk PM, Glynn JR 2008 Systematic review exploring time trends in the association between educational attainment and risk of HIV infection in sub-Saharan Africa. AIDS 22(3):403-14

75. Al-Taiar A, Chandler C, Al Eryani S, Whitty CJ

2009 Knowledge and practices for preventing severe malaria in Yemen: the importance of gender in planning policy. Health Policy and Planning 24(6):428-37

76. Girma1 B, Berhane Y 2011 Children who were vaccinated, breast fed and from low parity mothers live longer: A community based case-control study in Jimma, Ethiopia. BMC Public Health11:197

77. Chuangchaiya S, Jangpatarapongsa K, Chootong P, Sirichaisinthop J, Sattabongkot J, Pattanapanyasat K, Chotivanich K, Troye-Blomberg M, Cui L, Udomsangpetch R 2010 Immune response to Plasmodium vivax has a potential to reduce malaria severity. Clinical and Experimental Immunology 160(2):233-9

78. Parra M, Liu X, Derrick SC, Yang A, Tian J, Kolibab K, Kumar S, Morris SL 2013 Molecular analysis of non-specific protection against murine malaria induced by BCG vaccination. PLoS One 8(7)

79. BCG Vaccine, Wikipedia

80. Arama C, Waseem S, Fernández C, Assefaw-Redda Y, You L, Rodriguez A, Radošević K, Goudsmit J, Kaufmann SH, Reece ST, Troye-Blomberg M 2012 A recombinant Bacille Calmette-Guérin construct expressing the Plasmodium falciparum circumsporozoite protein enhances dendritic cell activation and primes for circumsporozoite-specific memory cells in BALB/c mice. Vaccine 30(37):5578-84

81. Teo WH, Nurul AA, Norazmi MN 2012 Immunogenicity of recombinant BCG-based vaccine expressing the 22 kDa of serine repeat antigen (SE22) of Plasmodium falciparum. Tropical Biomedicine 29(2):239-53

82. Rapeah S, Dhaniah M, Nurul AA, Norazmi MN 2010 Phagocytic activity and pro-inflammatory cytokines production by the murine macrophage cell line J774A.1 stimulated by a recombinant

BCG (rBCG) expressing the MSP1-C of Plasmodium falciparum. Tropical Biomedicine 27(3):461-9